V O I C E S *of*
A L Z H E I M E R ' S

VOICES *of* ALZHEIMER'S

Courage, Humor, Hope, and Love in the Face of Dementia

BETSY PETERSON

Da Capo
LIFE
LONG

A Member of the Perseus Books Group

Designed by Lisa Krienbrink
Set in 12 point Adobe Garamond Pro by The Perseus Books Group

Library of Congress Cataloging-in-Publication Data
Peterson, Betsy.
    Voices of Alzheimer's : courage, humor, hope, and love in the face of dementia / Betsy Peterson.
        p.   cm.
    Includes bibliographical references.
    ISBN 0-7382-0962-7 (pbk. : alk. paper)
    1. Alzheimer's disease—Anecdotes.
2. Alzheimer's disease—Humor.   3. Alzheimer's disease—Popular works.   I. Title.
    RC523.2.P485   2004
    362.196'831—dc22

2004015586

Published by Da Capo Press
A Member of the Perseus Books Group
http://www.dacapopress.com

Da Capo Press books are available at special discounts for bulk purchases in the U.S. by corporations, institutions, and other organizations. For more information, please contact the Special Markets Department at the Perseus Books Group, 11 Cambridge Center, Cambridge, MA 02142, or call (800) 255–1514 or (617) 252–5298, or email special.markets@perseusbooks.com.

1 2 3 4 5 6 7 8 9—08 07 06 05 04

Bare your wound,
let its voice instruct us
when we are afraid, telling us
not only of survival and pain, but
of courage and resistance, what it is
to be wounded yet whole.

—Marguerite Guzmán Bouvard,
from "Giving Testimony," *Wind, Frost & Fire*

Contents

Quotations

Contents

Contents

Foreword

*E*ach person bearing the diagnosis of Alzheimer's and each care partner orchestrating daily living offers a unique glimpse into the many faces of Alzheimer's. The ability to care for another being is based on personal traits of character, previous history with the patient, finances, community resources, and a host of other variables. Literature should be underscoring these unique qualities of our humanness by letting readers "hear" many varied voices. And yet, the literature seldom reflects this uniqueness. There are excellent books of advice and clinical dialogue, as well as books of individual reflection, but nothing that offers the varying ideas, differing opinions, and the roller-coaster emotions of living with dementia, in a format helpful to *all* patients, loved ones, and healthcare professionals.

Enter Betsy Peterson—a writer, lawyer, survivor, and active participant in life. Betsy was a care partner for her beloved husband, Pete, for fourteen years before he died. Drawing on her own unique experience and voices heard in other venues—support groups, conferences, workshops, conversations with friends, books, the Internet, and interviews—Betsy has created a powerfully helpful book to fill the void in the literature. Like Betsy herself, *Voices of Alzheimer's* is warm, witty, and wonderful.

Much knowledge about medications to control symptoms, differing but related diseases, and the pathology of the disease has evolved since Betsy began her care-partnering years. This has led families to at last have hope about finding a cure or at least halting the progression of Alzheimer's in their lifetime. The theme of hope resonates within these pages. Regardless of your relation to Alzheimer's disease, I find it hard to imagine not feeling enriched by the collected wisdom herein.

JOANNE KOENIG COSTE, M.ED., AUTHOR,
LEARNING TO SPEAK ALZHEIMER'S

Preface

$\mathcal{W}$hat is it like to live with Alzheimer's? Whether we are patients, family members, friends, or professionals, living with progressive memory loss and dementia is an experience that many of us find hard to talk about, even to ourselves.

This book breaks the silences between those who live with Alzheimer's—or another disease that causes similar brain damage—and those who don't. We complain that other people don't understand what Alzheimer's is like, but how can they understand if we can't tell them?

There was so much I couldn't talk about during my husband's illness, even to those willing to listen. My husband "Pete" was diagnosed with "probable Alzheimer's" in 1987. As his illness progressed, I felt increasingly lonely, as I was drawn into a separate world that had less and less connection to the other world I lived in. In the familiar, "normal" world, I went to work and did my shopping and chatted with friends and colleagues. But my Alzheimer's world was one they could barely imagine, even if they knew of Pete's illness. I didn't often try to explain it: it was too painful or private, or just made me feel more isolated. A friend might, for example, complain that her husband almost forgot their anniversary, but I would not mention that my husband could not tell you the names of his children. I could not share the little triumphs when we managed something tricky, like getting him a haircut, which became frightening for him, or the funny-but-painful moments like the time I found Pete using his toothbrush to brush his hair. It was lonely at home as Pete lost conversational skills, and it was lonely to be living in an Alzheimer's world so unfamiliar to my friends. Yet it took me almost seven years to admit that Alzheimer's is too hard to do alone, and to join the Alzheimer's community that was waiting to help. For me, as for many, joining a support group made all the difference in the world.

There, as in this book, I heard many voices and many moods. We could talk honestly about the hard parts; we could share "foxhole" laughter and ease the loneliness. All of us, whether patients or those who loved them, were unwilling explorers in the strange new world of dementia. We struggled to find our way through a landscape that is always changing and to adjust to a "new normal" again and again. But at least we could compare notes with others coping with such variables and get reports from the scouts who had gone before us. We became teachers and guides for each other as well as travel companions.

That's where I found courage, humor, hope, and love in the face of dementia. Not hope of a cure—at that time, there was no such hope, although there is now. But hope that I could find better ways to care for Pete and that future stages might in some ways be easier. Hope that I could learn to enjoy the happiness in my life and not just lament my sorrows.

If you live with dementia, as a patient or a family member or a friend, I hope the stories and insights in this book will help you connect, across the miles, with others facing a similar challenge. If you work with dementia as part of your job, I hope it will give you a larger sense of our experience. I hope too that this book will help bridge the gap between those who live with dementia and those who don't.

Yet the book tells us more than that. It's by people who have learned to live with Alzheimer's, despite the illness and because of it, coming to terms with the hardships and finding the treasures hidden in this new and different world. It is a book about life itself.

The Peterson Story

*O*f course every illness has its own unique mix of experiences. Our story is unique, but little of it is unusual.

My husband, Frederick A. Peterson, better known as "Pete," was diagnosed with "probable Alzheimer's" in the fall of 1987, at the age of seventy-one. At the time, he was busily enjoying retirement, and I was working as a lawyer for a publishing company.

We had been friends for many years before we married. When we met, Pete had been teaching for many years at Phillips Academy in Andover, Massachusetts. In 1966, he was in his second year as director of the Andover Summer Session, an enrichment program for students from all over the country. He decided he needed a year-round assistant and hired me—a daring step! Andover was still a boys' school and the Summer Session had been coeducational for only two years. During my three years in that job, his wife, Lee, and I also became good friends. Their eldest child, Rob, was away at school, but the young ones, Nancy Lee and John, accepted me as a sort of honorary aunt. The friendships continued when I moved to my next job, as an assistant dean of Yale College during the first years of undergraduate coeducation there. We exchanged visits back and forth and enjoyed vacations on the same lake in Maine. In the fall of 1975 I moved to Berkeley, California, to enter law school. That winter, Lee was diagnosed with lung cancer that had already spread. She died two years later.

Almost as soon as I returned to Boston after graduating from law school, Pete asked me to marry him. We planned the wedding while I was studying for the bar exam, and we were married on August 20, 1978.

Pete was sixty-two, and I was forty, but those who knew Pete worried whether I could keep up with him, not the other way around. He was a man of many interests and great enthusiasms. Some of these lasted only a few years—figure skating, vegetable gardening, learning Greek so he could read Homer. But Lee used to say that Pete had three passions that endured: teaching, sailing, and herself. It was my great good fortune to become the fourth.

Pete had been a teacher all his adult life, except for service in the navy during World War II. He taught English at Andover for thirty-nine years and made his students write every day, even if only a paragraph or two. He didn't read the newspaper at breakfast: he marked papers. He put that kind of dedication, attention, and persistence into any project he took seriously, along with excellent organizational skills, but it was his humor and zest that really distinguished his leadership style.

When Pete retired in 1981, we moved from Andover into Boston. He rejoiced in the flexibility of retirement—more time to read whatever he chose, more time to spend on our beloved Maine lake, and lots of time to enjoy living in the city for the first time. He thrived as a volunteer, in our neighborhood, on our lake, and for the Day Sailer Association. After a few years, however, we began to notice odd gaps in his memory and thought we should check them out. He made an appointment with a neurologist, but we weren't worried enough for me to take time off from work to go with him. That first visit in the fall of 1987 was generally reassuring—no brain tumor, only a recommendation that he find other people to pick up the leadership roles in his various activities.

The next summer we were making plans to gather family and close friends to join us at the lake to celebrate our tenth anniversary. This was just the kind of project Pete had always relished and performed with charm and efficiency. But this time he kept losing track of relatively simple arrangements. It didn't seem quite like forgetting, but as if the memories had never been made. So we made another appointment with the same neurologist, and this time we both went.

Some months later we sought a second opinion from the Memory Disorders Clinic at Massachusetts General Hospital. Both gave the same diagnosis: "probable Alzheimer's."

It was still hard to believe. Pete was so full of energy and enthusiasms—and so fit and good-looking—that most people thought he was in his fifties, not seventy-two. The diagnosis was never very far from my consciousness, and somehow I both believed and disbelieved it at the same time. It is hard to come to terms with a diagnosis that begins with "possible" or "probable," and there were many days when Pete seemed entirely his old self. For years almost nobody guessed anything was wrong. It was months before I told anybody outside the family, partly because it was so hard to imagine this lively, charming, intelligent man losing those gifts. But also, we didn't know much about Alzheimer's then. I vaguely remembered hearing that the movie star Rita Hayworth had gone into seclusion because of Alzheimer's, but that was it. I was afraid people would treat Pete strangely if they knew and would think he was "demented" in the popular sense. Alzheimer's was not yet a household word and not yet the not-so-secret fear of everyone over fifty.

In the beginning, most of the problems were relatively simple. We'd miss a social engagement because Pete forgot to tell me about a telephone call, or he'd promise to cook dinner and forget to shop. I was impatient and irritable; I kept thinking he could do better if he tried harder. It was years before I stopped wondering whether Pete would get better if he got a hearing aid or gave up alcohol. (We experimented with both.)

My loneliness began right away. My friends didn't know because I didn't tell them. Worse, Pete and I could seldom talk about it with each other. We had a few important discussions, but I cannot honestly say we faced the disease together. We made the journey side by side, but in very different and rather solitary ways.

What was it like for Pete? For the most part, I can only guess. Like many men of his generation, he was not in the habit of talking about painful feelings. And talking with him about Alzheimer's was complicated by two other circumstances. Pete did not usually remember he'd had the diagnosis, so mentioning it was like giving him bad news all over again. When we did speak of Alzheimer's, he mixed it up with Parkinson's and foresaw the progressive physical disability he'd witnessed in a colleague.

For Pete, I think the beginning was the most difficult phase. He was aware that he wasn't functioning as well as he had and would swear at himself for "being stupid." That was hard for both of us, and explaining that he had a medical problem causing memory loss didn't seem to help. But forgetting the diagnosis was also a gift: it spared Pete the depression and anxiety so many dementia patients suffer.

Some things got better as the disease got worse. After a few years, Pete seemed to lose his awareness of previous skills. In that respect, life became much easier for both of us. In fact, in those years I often thought Pete was one of the happiest people I had ever known—loving his family, finding much to enjoy in life, welcoming help, and no longer worrying about the past or the future. I admired that contentment and could sometimes share it, but on the whole, I was worrying a lot more than before.

For many years, Pete was able to use his intelligence to maneuver around his memory problems. He enjoyed friends and family and being outdoors and messing about in boats. Slowly, slowly, however, the dementia took a greater toll. Pete started getting lost when he went out for a drive or a walk, and he eventually became dependent on others to get anywhere or to be safe at home. I kept on working, although I eventually shifted to part-time, but the day-to-day complications became more and more demanding. I would find myself late for work because it took longer than usual to get Pete ready for the day; I would hurry home leaving work unfinished when I knew he was alone. In other ways, too, it was something like being the single parent of a young child, but without the hope that he would grow out of it. Pete was going to need more help as time went on, not less.

Despite the complications and the losses, it wasn't all gloom and doom. We had some wonderful trips, although these became easier if a friend came along with us. Visits with the family were always fun, although it was poignant when Pete began to prefer the grandchildren's games to the adult activities. We had always found it magical to spend time at our camp on the lake in Maine, and we treasured it even more keenly now. In the past, Pete had thrown himself into energetic projects. He ran the sailing races and the lake environmental association; he loved chopping wood and rowing miles in his racing shell. Now he would spend long stretches of time sitting on the dock or the porch. That bothered me until I realized how actively he was watching the ever-changing light and motion on the water or in the woods. Instead of sculling his racing shell, he spent hours joyfully puttering about in our little dinghy. He became more contemplative, whereas I became busier and more outgoing. As I lost the old pleasures of Pete's conversation and companionship at home, I had to reach out to make new friends, and I found them—in a book group, at church, and in an Alzheimer's support group.

Although Pete's verbal skills held out for a long time, social life became a challenge. I had never realized how much of our normal social chitchat consists of asking questions until my husband was unable to answer routine inquiries about the children or a recent vacation. It wasn't unusual for him to tell the same story three times within a few minutes, or repeat a question again and again, or make it embarrassingly clear that he wanted to go home. As the illness progressed, he found social settings more and more confusing, which gave every outing a new unpredictability and tension.

There were rough moments and many puzzles. If he became upset, those of us who knew him well could usually understand what had upset him—too sudden a gesture, too long a wait, too much going on. But as the illness deepened, I felt so often a sense of mystery, especially when Pete no longer had any words. I remember one day in particular, when we tried to leave our daughter's house. Pete would not get off the sofa. We let him be for twenty minutes before trying again, which was often a successful tactic, but the second attempt failed, and the third, and the fourth, and however many more. I went through my entire repertoire of strategies without success. He didn't seem agitated, or afraid, or even tired, but he didn't budge. Why, why? Somehow, two hours later, Nancy Lee persuaded him to stand up. By then I was sobbing, out of sight in the hallway. I got our coats, and we led him gently to the door and into the car. What was he experiencing that made it so hard for him that day?

And what is it like to be an adult who cannot speak? Did Pete still think in words? How much of our words did he understand? We tried to act as if he understood, and often I believed he did—only to feel a few minutes later that my words had no meaning for him. But even then it seemed clear that the *sounds* had meaning: he would react to tone and feeling whether or not he understood the words as words.

Eventually Pete's vocabulary dwindled to an idiosyncratic "be-be-be." Some people thought this syllable was a remnant of "Betsy," and I liked to think so. There had been a phase when he had lost most of his vocabulary but would often say, "Betsy, Betsy, Betsy, I love you." And then one day I realized I hadn't heard that for weeks. It was one of those non-events that marks a profound change.

We were lucky in many ways. Pete usually enjoyed social interaction, even as he lost language. His sense of humor and his sweetness— and his need to exert his own will—endured almost to the very end. I rarely had to deal with difficult behaviors such as wandering, violence, or catastrophic responses. Neither of us had other notable health problems, most of the time. We both escaped serious depression. We had enough money to buy services—help at home, a day program, assisted living. Once I got over trying to do it alone, I had excellent support—from family and friends, from a support group and a superb local chapter of the Alzheimer's Association, from the people who came to help us at home and those who staffed the day program and the assisted living center. In particular, our daughter, Nancy Lee, was always ready to listen or pitch in and to share difficult decisions. It could have been much harder.

For better and for worse, however, Pete's illness progressed very slowly. In 1987, when he was diagnosed, the conventional prediction was that patients typically survive for another four to seven years. In our case, it was seven years before I admitted that the time had come to seek out a day program for him and a regular support group for me. It was twelve years before I gave up taking care of him at home. When he died, nearly fourteen years after diagnosis, he had outlived almost all the other participants in a large study researching the long-term course of the disease.

In January 1999, some things suddenly got much harder; for example, I could no longer count on getting his clothes off before he went to bed or on getting him out of bed in the morning. He had a short bout with some virus and seemed sometimes just too tired to send to the day program. I was exhausted and finally admitted that the dreaded time had come. We knew he would do best in a specialized Alzheimer's unit. By the time we made the decision, I had visited nine or ten. In February, Nancy Lee and I took the excruciating step of moving Pete into residential care at one of the many facilities run by a company called Sunrise Assisted Living.

Moving Pete away from home felt worse than a death—and as if I had to be the executioner. But at the time I told only our closest family and friends that we were taking this step, and I went to work as usual the next day. There are no social conventions or religious rituals to mark that sad transition.

Within a few months, I had settled into the odd routine of seeing my husband only two or three times a week, driving an hour each way. Pete and the Sunrise staff and I became comfortable with each other. Thank God, because in the fall of 2000, I learned that I had breast cancer. It would not have been possible to manage both his illness and mine at home.

The cancer story started simply—I didn't even have a lump—but it got more complicated at every step. I ended up having a lung biopsy first, to make sure an unidentifiable spot in my lung was not a metastasis (it wasn't), then a mastectomy, and then chemotherapy. I was on medical leave from my job for four months.

Pete was too sick to understand that I had cancer, and I didn't try to tell him. It was a very strange winter for me. Sometimes I couldn't get to see Pete for a week or two, and suddenly most of the attention—including mine—was on my own health. Friends and family rallied wonderfully to help me through the long months of treatment. But the contrast between dealing with cancer and living with Alzheimer's was stunning.

Part of that was purely medical. My cancer was discovered early, and after following well-established treatment protocols, I have a very good chance it won't recur. For Alzheimer's, however, there is still no cure. During most of Pete's illness, there weren't even medications to relieve symptoms. (Several are available now.) But everything else was different too. There was no ambiguity about my own diagnosis, no "probable" about the presence of cancer cells. The news was bad, but the clarity was almost a relief. And suddenly the medical world was there to help us out. As a cancer patient, the doctors offered me encouragement and choices of treatment, not the dispiriting resignation that marked our discussions of dementia. Moreover, our health insurance covered almost all my cancer expenses, although it provided almost nothing for Pete's Alzheimer's care.

Even more striking, however, was the social context. Many people have learned how to help and encourage a cancer patient. I got flowers, cards, prayers, phone calls, casseroles. These were wonderfully welcome but would have been even more precious during my caregiving years—especially the casseroles.

Then, just as I was finishing chemotherapy, Pete got some kind of infection. We arranged for hospice care to supplement the staff at Sunrise. He died there three weeks later, on April 20, 2001, at sunset.

The next week, and his memorial service in the school chapel at Andover, brought a mixture of sorrow, relief, and exhaustion—but also, to my surprise, joy. Family, friends, and former colleagues and students shared their love of this man and gave new life to happy memories that had faded during his illness. The service included many of Pete's enthusiasms: trumpet and organ, Chaucer and Robert Frost, funny stories as well as hymns and tributes. It ended with the Royal Fireworks Music—his choice. Best of all were the cherry blossoms. Over many years, Pete had raised the money for more than a hundred cherry trees around the school campus and planted most of them himself. Somehow, despite the fickle weather that week, they were in full and glorious bloom.

Months later, Pete's story had a surprise ending. We had, with some discomfort, donated his brain to Massachusetts General Hospital. We had never questioned Pete's diagnosis of Alzheimer's, which had been made by two of the best memory disorder clinics in the country, but we felt it important to honor Pete's earlier decision to contribute to research as much as he could. When the report finally came, eight months after his death, I was stunned. He had not had Alzheimer's. There were only a few of the plaques and neurofibrillary tangles that mark Alzheimer's, so his brain tissue did not meet the criteria for that disease. Instead, the neuropathological findings were "consistent with the features of the group of diseases called frontotemporal dementias." The pathologist did not venture an opinion on which of those frontotemporals it might be. In short, Pete had been the victim of a disease that was an even bigger medical mystery than Alzheimer's.

It took a while to get over the shock of redefining the past fourteen years. I usually still tell people that Pete had Alzheimer's—partly because it's a term more people understand, and partly because I hate the word dementia. Everybody thought we were living with Alzheimer's, and so we did. The similarities were far more profound than the differences. There was no lost opportunity for treatment: no medications have yet been proven helpful for frontotemporal dementias.

And yet the differences matter. I realized after getting the autopsy report that the experience would have been even lonelier if we had known he had a rare disease. It was a comfort as well as a tragedy to have had so much company with Alzheimer's. It had been a comfort to follow the exciting progress toward treating Alzheimer's, even though the new medications were coming too late to help Pete. There was even a piece of probable good news: there is less likelihood of a genetic link, and thus less risk for his children. But beyond all that? I can almost hear Pete chuckling—the teacher is still teaching, and the experts still have much to learn.

And Pete is still teaching me. I learned so much from him, and also from his illness, and then from putting together this book.

I had been brooding, all during the cancer treatment, about quitting my job. I was sixty-two. I could take early retirement but was scared to leave without some new focus. I'd begun to think about this book, and I was learning so much from the contrast between the cancer and Alzheimer's experiences. Could these misfortunes help me to help others? I applied to a program for people working on independent projects, the Scholars Program of the Women's Studies Research Center at Brandeis University.

Then, one crucial week in April, Pete died, and I was invited to join the Scholars for one year as a visiting research associate. I didn't hesitate. These were the signals to quit my job and start a new chapter. This was a change I could choose.

The Scholars Program was great. I began to work on the book, in spurts amidst other projects. Life was full of activities I enjoyed—seminars, volunteer work, friends, and family. At last I had a grandchild within driving distance, Megan, newly adopted from China.

Becoming a full-fledged widow, however, was much more confusing and time-consuming than I expected. I thought I'd had enough practice—I'd lived alone for two years and handled all financial and household matters for much longer. This was oddly different. I missed Pete in new ways. I kept wishing we could enjoy all these blessings together. My life felt like scattered pieces of a jigsaw puzzle, not a picture.

Gradually, and with help, I began to understand that these transitions were going to take years, not months. Gradually, too, I learned that my task was not to "let go" of Pete, but to redefine that relationship. It would continue to change for the rest of my life, just as it had changed in the years before, as we went from colleagues to friends to husband and wife. The losses had started years before Pete's death, but the bonds had held then and continue still.

And all those years with Pete were such an extraordinary gift. There was a moment, a few years into Pete's illness, when a school classmate I hadn't seen for years was lamenting that we had been married only nine years when Pete was diagnosed. I found myself protesting, "But I'm still way ahead!"

That is still true. I have had the treasure of a really good marriage—for better and for worse, in sickness and in health. Yes, of course there were times when I could only feel sorry for myself, but our marriage was such a blessing and its rewards continue. One day, looking at a family photo, I realized with a sudden jolt, "Good heavens, I've become a matriarch!" Pete's family is now mine too. It has been a privilege to become a second mother to his three children and a grandmother to six.

It's that overriding blessing—Pete's love and loving Pete—that got me through the hard parts of his illness and sustains me still. Now, three years after Pete's death, I think I am in one of the happiest phases of my life and one of the happiest people I know. Cancer and

Alzheimer's have helped me cherish life, even its mixtures of joy and pain. The work of this book has been a mixture too. It has been hard to spend so much time revisiting the pain of Alzheimer's. But it is a cherished privilege to make deeper and wider connections with others who have faced that pain and to learn from their courage, humor, hope, and love.

Notes to Reader

If you've met one family with Alzheimer's, you've met one family with Alzheimer's.

Lisa Gwyther, MSW, Education Director,
Bryan Alzheimer's Disease Research Center, Duke University

*A*nd each person in each family has a different perspective and experience. My comments are in italics, usually at the end of a section. Everyone else is identified by his or her relationship to the disease: as a patient, or as the spouse or child or friend of a person with dementia.

I've drawn these quotations from many sources. I heard many of the "voices" firsthand in conversations with my friends or in support groups or other Alzheimer's gatherings. Others come from books, broadcasts, and the Internet. Some quotations are from professional writers: novelists Jonathan Franzen and Sue Miller, sports commentator and journalist Charles Pierce, and literary critic John Bayley, husband of the novelist Iris Murdoch. There are two famous patients, former president Ronald Reagan and the nineteenth-century philosopher and writer Ralph Waldo Emerson.

Most of the comments, however, are from people who became writers or gave speeches only because they found themselves living with dementia. The Sources section in the back of the book gives profiles of some of these contributors and information on the published sources.

Caution! Each quotation in this book is only one person's report, from one point in time and a particular set of circumstances. Many comments do express a response that I've heard from many patients or family members. But I have also tried to suggest the incredible variability of living with dementia.

One of the hardest things about living with Alzheimer's or any other dementia is the unpredictability. You can study the lists of symptoms and definitions of stages, but no one—not even the most skilled clinician—can predict whether or when the person you love will, for example, start to wander or refuse to bathe or have hallucinations. These are not unusual problems, but many patients never experience these symptoms.

It isn't just that dementia affects one patient differently from another with the same diagnosis and that the symptoms change over time. It can affect the same person differently from day to day, sometimes from one moment to the next. And so our responses vary enormously too—not just from one person to another, and not just over time, but within ourselves from day to day and moment to moment.

Some Language Issues

Alzheimer's, dementia. Technically, Alzheimer's is only one of many diseases that cause dementia, although it is by far the most common. The medical world defines "dementia" as deterioration of intellectual faculties, such as memory, concentration, and judgment, resulting from an organic disease or disorder of the brain.

As a practical matter, the differences between Alzheimer's and other dementias don't matter nearly as much to the patient and family and friends as the core similarity, the progressive loss of cognitive functions. Even the experts often use the term "Alzheimer's"—now a household word—to include similar diseases.

Many families, including ours, avoid the word "dementia," even when it's not Alzheimer's. For some, that's because so many lay people use the word "demented" to describe crazy behavior, which many patients never display. Or, in the words of patient Gloria Sterin:

I have a memory problem, but I don't think I am demented. Dementia means I don't have a mind. There's something very degrading about that word. I'd like to see it done away with.

Patient. Some people have trouble deciding what to call people who suffer from the disease. "Person with dementia" is perhaps the most neutral term, but it's too clumsy for use in most of this book. I have chosen "patient" because the root meaning of the word is very fitting: it comes from a Latin verb meaning to suffer, to endure.

Caregiver, care partner. "Caregiver" has been the term traditionally applied to family and friends caring for a dementia patient. (It may also refer to people paid for such work, such as nursing home staff.) A recent trend is to refer to family members as "care partners" rather than "caregivers," especially in the early stages of the illness. For me, however, the term "caregiver" was an important part of a slow but necessary redefinition of my relationship to Pete—the transition to seeing ourselves as "patient" and "caregiver" as well as husband and wife.

Quotations

Something's Wrong

It's very difficult for a person with Alzheimer's to experience his disease. You cannot experience what you have forgotten.

JIM ANTHONY, *patient*

I felt different, like I was changing. Things just didn't work as smoothly.

RUTH HARRIS, *patient*

I became lost while driving over familiar roads near home. I feared I had suffered a stroke.

CATHLEEN MCBRIDE, *patient*

My wife and kids seemed to be constantly angry with me for telling the "wrong" joke or flirting with someone too much. I had to ask my wife to come with me to doctors' appointments because I would get there and forget what I wanted to say.

JOHN DURAND, *patient*

I took early retirement because of memory problems, but with relief—I had been worrying for some time about making calamitous mistakes due to my memory problems. Then I volunteered to edit a monthly newsletter. Initially, it took me about three days; two years later, I could not finish a newsletter before the next was due. It seemed the end of being human to me, and I rapidly became very depressed and seriously thought of suicide. I finally got an MRI scan, which did not show anything amiss. One neuropsychologist suggested I was malingering. I really blew my top!

LEWIS LAW, *patient*

I understand now what happened but all I knew then was that something was very wrong. As time went on, this same problem began to show up in many situations . . . while driving, in the crowded cafeteria at work, crowded grocery store, etc. I eventually came to understand that my periods of "lost time" occurred when I was in a situation where there were too many stimuli for my brain to handle, and it would tune out everything happening around me until it could catch up with all the input it had received. This would result in me being aware of where I was and what I was doing at point A in time and place and then suddenly becoming aware of myself and surroundings again at point C in time and place . . . but with no ability at all to retrieve the memory of what had happened between A and C.

DOREEN, *patient, Pick's disease*

Doggone, I never thought I'd lose my *mind.*
JAMES NICHOLS, *patient, realizing he had "seen" small children when none were present*

* * *

For a long time, I thought that my mom was forgetful, easily irritated, and pretty ornery—more than usual, but not discontinuous from who she was. We were planning a party for her and decided not to make it a surprise party because we didn't want to shock her. So we told her about the party, planned the invitations with her, and talked about it on the way to the restaurant. When we got there, and she saw the guests, her face lit up, and she thanked us exuberantly for giving her this surprise party. Finally, two and two made four and I knew she had some form of dementia.

MARSHA, *daughter*

She's served me pizza every night for six months.

JOE, husband

She wrote a check for $500 when it was supposed to be $5. You think, "I can't believe this." It's not only what's happening and their memory, it's the feeling of "*I don't know what to do now.*"

MAUREEN, daughter

I felt Dad might be telling me, in essence, that it was none of my damned business. Maybe that was true, I don't know. Certainly I was always able to shift quickly to thinking so, to feeling as guilty for trying to do something as for doing nothing—because while I didn't want to be irresponsible, I didn't want to be intrusive either.

SUE MILLER, daughter

We were in trouble long before the diagnosis. I couldn't understand why my husband's business seemed to be going downhill. When he failed to do something he'd promised to do, I thought he was not paying attention or didn't care for me any more, and I took it personally. We became very unhappy with each other years before guessing he had a medical problem.

CARLA, wife

Something's Wrong

Felicity's early signs were depression and fender benders, and she wasn't yet sixty. It didn't occur to me that her problem might be dementia. My denial overrode my training as a physician.

DANIEL, *husband*

I remembered Thanksgiving, my father refusing to take his coat off, and insisting from the time he came up the stairs that he had to go home. But you haven't had dinner yet, I told him. Oh, he replied. Then, he would make for the door again. You can't walk home, I'd say. It's too far. Oh, he replied.

I'd seen it and not seen it. Instead, I had asked my mother if he'd ever done anything like this before, and she said, no, never, and I believed her.

CHARLES PIERCE, *son*

We just got word from an excellent memory specialist that my husband's most recent tests do not show any problem. That should be good news, but we both know something is wrong. Now we have to prove it!

GLADYS, *wife*

I am nearly beside myself with frustration. By now, we've been to our primary physician, and a neurologist, and a psychiatrist, and my wife has taken a variety of tests. Sometimes she does pretty well at those, but at work she can't even put papers in alphabetical order. The company is willing to set up disability pay, but I can't get any of those doctors to give us the documentation.

KURT, *husband*

Certainly I saw his oddness, when he was odd, more sharply than my siblings. But even I didn't really want to confront it. It came and went anyway, and so again and again I was able to argue myself out of acknowledging it.

SUE MILLER, *daughter*

In some ways the beginning was the hardest part—when Bill was still working and we were pretending things were all right. Once people knew he had a medical problem, it was a lot easier.

CAROL, *wife*

❦

One Christmas, Pete gave us both a neat present—windbreakers especially designed for rowers, with long tails and nothing to catch your hands on. When the ice finally went out of our lake and I brought them out again, Pete exclaimed with surprise. It was as if he had never seen them before—no memory of choosing them as a special present, no memory that I had been delighted by the gift. I began to understand that his memory loss was quite different from the forgetfulness I had seen in other older people.

Diagnosis

I'd known something was going wrong for at least three years, even though another doctor, two years before, had told me everything was normal. It was a great relief to get the diagnosis.

I had more tests than I can remember, and they all seemed to indicate Alzheimer's. Alzheimer's cannot be precisely diagnosed until the patient is dead. I try to be cooperative with my health care givers, but there are simply some things I will not do for medical science.

JIM ANTHONY, *patient*

That doctor was so rude. He wouldn't tell me the names of the last four presidents.

MILLICENT, *patient*

Damn it all. Am I invisible? This is *my* disease you're talking about—I'm still here. Talk to me. Me!

> JASON, *patient (When the doctor gave the diagnosis of Alzheimer's, he initially addressed the patient's wife. The doctor apologized and then directed his remarks to Jason.)*

I felt some relief. At first, I was grateful that I didn't have something more life-threatening, such as a brain tumor. I also felt a real fear for the future for myself and my family, although I already knew my wife, Carol, is a brilliant coper.

> BILL ORME-JOHNSON, *patient*

The first neuropsychologist criticized my "inappropriate flirting" and "inappropriate joking" during the examination. I was furious when she told me she was going to give me a test to rule out malingering. She concluded that all of my symptoms were related to my depression. My wife and I were confused and upset. Eventually, the hospital "rewrote" my evaluation, from depression to frontal temporal dementia. Eventually we changed hospitals and neurologists.

> JOHN DURAND, *patient*

Diagnosis

Oh, my dear, you're going to have one hell of a time.
> HOWARD CAREW *to his wife, upon his diagnosis*

I threw away my conservative clothes when I got the diagnosis. Life is too serious—now I wear a polo shirt with Mickey Mouse on it.
> FRANK CARLINO, *patient*

Getting this news is not fun, and it does not make me happy, but it sure as hell beats getting run over by a car without being prepared. Now I can get on with living for whatever time is left.
> BILL, *patient*

The most challenging issue is that the doctors still won't give a diagnosis, except that it's some kind of memory problem. One has to live with an undetermined future: total uncertainty.
> LEWIS LAW, *patient*

✦   ✦   ✦

The reality is that even a diagnosis doesn't help with planning. The doctors can only tell you that Alzheimer's patients may live from two to twenty years after diagnosis, and they know even less about other dementias.

RUTH GORDON, *support group leader*

We thought it was so hard not to have a firm diagnosis. But then we got results from a PET scan, which our doctor felt were conclusive. It eliminated all the "maybes," and that was hard too. You have to take it in steps.

MARY, *wife*

In the beginning it was like somebody hit you over the head with a baseball bat, you know, you don't want to believe it, and I think you close your eyes to it too. After the initial shock, I tended not even to think about it.

JILL, *wife*

It took us a good six months to tell my husband's daughter. We just had to come to the realization ourselves before we could talk with family members. We had to accept it for ourselves before we could explain it to others.

CORINNE, *wife*

It was real. It could be named. It was Alzheimer's disease. And I felt my guilty relief to know it . . . mixed, of course, with real sorrow for Dad. But the diagnosis signaled the end to the nameless anxiety that I felt had been mine alone for years, and for that, no matter what, I was grateful.

SUE MILLER, *daughter*

One of the neurologists pointed out the five realities we had to live with, even though they could not at that time give a name to Jim's condition (later defined as PSP, a rare dementia). Jim's condition was organic, neurological, progressive, degenerative, and untreatable.

Organic: it was physical, beyond Jim's control. That word was an enormous relief.

Neurological: involves all body systems and has major consequences for all.

Progressive: likely to change constantly (usually right after we figured out the previous change).

Degenerative: a growing series of losses.

Incurable: although it can be managed.

PAM KUNKEMUELLER, *wife*

Understanding the diagnosis was hard. We cried a lot and yelled at each other. "I understand it all," Julian eventually said. "I know where I'm headed. But let's be happy in the rest of my life." His words cut off my anger. They challenged me to accept this tough reality and reframe my grief.

ANN DAVIDSON, *wife*

Don't feel you have to learn everything about Alzheimer's immediately. You need to monitor your own intake. There's a lot of stuff in the books that may never happen to you or the one you love.

NANCY KING, *a previous director of Alzheimer's Association, Massachusetts Chapter*

One of the most helpful things anybody said? "You didn't cause it, and you won't cure it."

DOROTHY, *wife*

❧

I kept telling myself that the neurologist's diagnosis did not change the present reality—that my husband was still loving, lovable, intelligent, full of joie de vivre and fun to be with despite the unpredictable lapses. But a few weeks later I read up on Alzheimer's. I scared myself silly and couldn't tell anyone for months. I couldn't share that fear with Pete, either. He seemed to have forgotten the diagnosis, and wouldn't it be cruel to remind him? It was a great relief when the news came out "accidentally" during a visit from two of our oldest friends. We needed their help to talk about it with each other.

Patients

People with memory problems aren't stupid. They are people with memory problems.

Patient

Alzheimer's is not a dirty word.

FRANK CARLINO, *patient*

This disease takes courage.

Patient

Life with dementia can be like a roller coaster ride blindfolded . . . you know there will be a lot of ups and downs, but you don't even know when you are going to get hit with them.

DOREEN, *patient*

I'm still here. Parts of me are missing, but parts of me are still damn good.

> *Patient*

You're not a gork, you're a person.

> TERRY, *patient*

I see it as a fog that imperceptibly becomes thicker. You don't notice the darkness until you realize that you cannot see. You try to carry on normally, but you stumble around and bark your shins on objects you cannot see.

> JIM ANTHONY, *patient*

Do I have the plague? I must, because no one will talk about what's happening to me. And if I ask about it, the subject is changed.

> *Patient*

At the moment I feel just fine. I will continue to share life's journey with my beloved Nancy and my family . . . I now begin the journey that will lead me into the sunset of my life.

> RONALD REAGAN, *patient, former president*

I keep a 3x5 card in my pocket with the words "It's not my fault" written on it. It's a reminder to me *and* my family.

BARNEY, *patient*

When I think about how I feel, it's not good, not terrible—it's no man's land.

Patient

People shouldn't dwell on the problems I have with some tasks. I need help with the successes.

MICHAEL, *patient*

The constant testing by family members enraged me.

BART, *patient*

I'm losing my mind—but the essence of a person is their heart. I hope as I grow older I'll still be able to laugh—and to hug—and to know love.

FRAN NOONAN POWERS, *patient*

It's like blank spaces in my mind. I know something—but it isn't there.

BUTCH NOONAN, patient

Listen to my feelings, not just my words.

Patient

To family members, I say, "Don't baby me, and don't pretend it isn't there." To friends, I say, "Let me talk about it sometimes. Whether I'm angry or sad, just listen."

JEAN, patient

My memory is impaired, not my intelligence.

CATHLEEN MCBRIDE, patient

Losing my mind is losing myself.

PETE, patient

If I get information slowly by one person, I stand a good chance of getting it right. If it's noisy, I can't untangle it.

AL, patient

Having Alzheimer's is like sucking pond water. If you don't learn to deal with it, you may drown.

STAN EVANS, *patient*

I was diagnosed at fifty-eight and decided to take early retirement. That meant an end to my life as I had known it. I felt, and still often feel, like I am no longer an adequate adult. And I was very angry—at my colleagues, at my diagnosis, and at how my life was changing. I had to give up many outside activities such as board memberships and some church activities. It was a real killer to have to admit to myself and to my family that I could no longer undertake those responsibilities.

BILL ORME-JOHNSON, *patient*

It took me a long time to let up on myself.

Patient

Once a disease is named, especially if it is Alzheimer's, you begin to understand it, and that means recognizing it in everyday things. It is not long before you are under the spell of the disease. I worry this disease in me will hijack my life with my permission.

THOMAS DEBAGGIO, *patient*

It is as if fewer thoughts ooze out, or they ooze more slowly. Or that I have less energy to think them or put them together.

MORRIS FRIEDELL, *patient*

If there is one thing that I want to impart to others, it is this: please remember how terrifying dementia can be. Those of us who have it are fearful every minute of every day, although we sometimes do not show it. We need a great deal of physical and emotional support to help us find and use all the brainpower that we still have.

BILL ORME-JOHNSON, *patient*

A friend of mine gave me a book on a woman who was writing about her Alzheimer's and how gloriously, wonderfully she was handling her disease. I hated that book. I wouldn't consider behaving as well as she did. I want to cry and whine and kick! I'm angry. I'm angry that anybody has it.

JEAN, *patient*

Primary Family Care Partners

I hate that Peggi is my caregiver now instead of my equal partner.

JOHN DURAND, *patient*

He's not my caregiver—he's my husband.

Patient

I only wish there was some way I could spare Nancy from this painful experience.

RONALD REAGAN, *patient, former president*

Poor Joe, he's stuck with me all of the time. I try to get him to go down and play pool for a few hours.

BEA, *patient*

Sometimes I give my wife a hard time just to be nasty. I guess it's because I'd like to be doing things myself instead of having someone telling me to do this or do that. I'm a little boy now. I have a mommy to take care of me. It's not a very good feeling.

BOB, *patient*

My wife wants to help me whether I need it or not. I want to say, "Don't help me unless I ask for it."

Patient

I've seen people become very angry with me and with other people with Alzheimer's, especially partners and family members. The reason, I suspect, is that Alzheimer's is very frightening. One prefers to think that his or her companion is simply not trying hard enough, is being careless, obstinate, difficult, even deliberately trying to provoke.

JIM ANTHONY, *patient*

We love each other. We have for fifty-five years, and that's not going to change.

BETTY, *patient*

It's good to be on the same page with your mate. So many times I don't connect. Out of nowhere I say something and expect my honey to jump right in and connect where my mind has wandered for the moment. When she finds where I am, I jump to some other thought. I want her to be a mind reader of sorts and not take too long in doing it, but yet not be too quick so that I don't have time to do it for myself.

I ask her for the impossible. Caregivers just can't please sometimes, no matter how hard they try.

CHIP GERBER, *patient*

. . .

It's a tough job.

CARL SCOVEL, *son and a minister, to a caregiver*

I take care of Hughes in order to be able to face and live with myself. I am not a martyr; I do this not so much for Hughes as for myself. I do this to be true to myself and to my beliefs.

LELA SHANKS, *wife*

She would do it for me.

CHRIS, *sister*

I need my husband to help me care for my husband, but I don't have him any more, even though he is still here.

ZINNIA, *wife*

Having been a caregiver for my mother and now for my husband, I think husband is easier. Why? A child is always trying to please and protect the parent. A spouse is a partner—a contemporary, and more comfortable to deal with and try to think for.

MARY, *daughter, wife*

My life? I was terrified all the time that the phone would ring.

JUNE, *daughter*

I understand that there is only one drug in the world that can keep my mother calm and contented, and I am that drug.

ELEANOR COONEY, *daughter*

Unfortunately, I never had a good relationship with my mother in the first place. That's made it tougher in some ways, but perhaps less of a sorrow.

LINDA, *daughter*

It was hard for me to become my mother's caregiver. I was the youngest, so I was pretty spoiled. To be a caregiver was very difficult for both of us. She didn't want the youngest kid telling her what to do, and as the youngest, I wanted to be out on my own.

GENNY MCGLYNN, *daughter*

One day when Mom was especially annoyed . . . she walked down the hall to the bathroom, and stood in front of the mirror. I could see her talking to her reflection . . . . A few minutes later she returned to me and said, "The lady in the bathroom is MUCH nicer than you are!"

JEANNE PARSONS, *daughter*

I didn't realize how angry many family members are until I went to that workshop. I think it's easier for me because I didn't know Jim before he was diagnosed.

BRUCE, *partner*

People simply don't value caregiving for someone who loses their thinking process. We caregivers tend to be characterized as victims, and our people tend to be characterized as burdensome because of this bias. I found that demoralizing.

BEVERLY BIGTREE MURPHY, *wife*

It's such a challenge to *always* be thinking for the two of us. There are many times I think Terry understands or remembers—I relax a little and then find out I had misread him.

MARY, *wife*

Caregiving as such is a process—an evolutionary process, a learning process. Caregivers are learners first. . . . Often it is not so much the tasks themselves as our resistance to them that causes us stress and wears us down.

LELA SHANKS, *wife*

You have to give yourself permission to not be perfect—you can't be. It's a big, unpredictable job.

EDNA BALLARD, *social worker,*
Duke University Alzheimer's Family Support Program

When I am tired and getting impatient about all the demands my wife puts on me, I try to treat her as if it were our last day together.

T. S., *husband*

Frankly, I find it quite peaceful to grapple with serious problems from time to time. Caregiving is actually a very good asana. Keeps one's chi flowing and the Tao open.

DAYIN

❦

The single thing I most wish I had done differently in those early years? Taken a whole summer off to enjoy with my husband. He was still well enough for us to enjoy many of the things we had loved doing together, but I could see the downward curve. I thought about taking a leave from my job. Now I wish that I had.

But keeping my job was the right choice for me, although I eventually shifted to working part-time. Of course there were times when the stress of the job and the stress at home made a terrible combination, but on the whole, the job and the daily routine and supportive colleagues helped me keep a balance I might easily have lost on my own. Economically, it made a lot more sense to keep earning a good salary than to lose it. It could pay for help at home and, later, for my husband to attend a day program.

The Rest of the Family

My sons are dealing with this very well. They are always joshing me, and it's fun. They used to learn from me, and now I have to learn from them. I don't really like it. I feel like it's topsy-turvy but that's the way it has to be.

BILL, *patient*

I can only guess what my wife, Joyce, and my son, Francesco, are going through. . . . Alzheimer's hit them as surely as it has hit me. They are reluctant to reveal their pain and fear to me, but every time they see me or talk to me they must be reminded of their own sorrow and fear. Although we try to avoid talking about Alzheimer's, I know it is on the edge of their thoughts every day, as it is mine.

THOMAS DeBAGGIO, *patient*

My children are sometimes very angry and hurt by things I've said or done. I never mean to hurt them. I am very proud that they have learned to be sensitive and loving toward me in spite of all this disease takes away from us. It is very difficult to know that I can no longer be the dad to them that I had always been.

JOHN DURAND, *patient with teenage children*

The part that drove me up the wall was knowing how hard it would be on my family—I had seen this with my brother-in-law—and that I could do nothing about it.

BART, *patient*

◆   ◆   ◆

It's not about us, the family. It's about them, the patients.

MAUREEN REAGAN, *daughter of Ronald Reagan*

It's about all of us. When a person has Alzheimer's, the whole family is enormously impacted.

MARSHA, *daughter*

Last summer I got laid off from my job—and it was such a blessing! I was able to spend a lot of time with my mother and give my dad a break. We'd go to the beach or just hang out together. I treasure the time we have been able to spend together.

Daughter

Dad mellowed in many ways that made us much closer. There had always been some tension between us. The disease took the edges off—but not all of them. He would blow up at me if I reached to help him up the stairs—but react gracefully when my wife, Lisa, did the same thing.

JOHN, *son*

Coming home had always meant a chance to refuel on my parents' nurturing. This time I found my father out of touch and my mother's energies absorbed in his care. The child in me was screaming, "This is not the way it's supposed to be!" I felt a sense of loss for both my mother and my father. . . . I was happy when the visit ended—relieved that we lived far away.

SHELA OMELL RICHARDS, *daughter*

Task by task, my mother took charge of their life. And so, although my father's "long illness" was a crushing disappointment to my mother, it was also an opportunity to grow slowly into an autonomy she'd never been allowed: to settle some very old scores.

As for me, once I accepted the scope of the disaster, the sheer duration of Alzheimer's forced me into unexpectedly welcome closer contact with my mother. I learned, as I might not have otherwise, that I could seriously rely on my brothers and that they could rely on me.

JONATHAN FRANZEN, *son*

My father cared for my mother all those years, at home. Day in and day out. I view his devotion as heroic . . . but my father saw this burden as an honor.

EDWARD MARKEY, *son, U.S. Congressman*

My mother is the one with the diagnosis, but my father is the victim. And yet I think there are ways in which he makes himself the victim—for example, by refusing our help.

KAREN, *daughter*

It's been hard to be so far away. I worry more about my father. My mother is in a nursing home now, and seems content, and is well taken care of, but I can scarcely imagine how hard it is for him. Cancer would be easier.

KIT, *daughter (and a cancer survivor)*

My dad hasn't said my name in probably two years, but he knows me because I'm the guy who hugs him.

MICHAEL REAGAN, *son of Ronald Reagan*

One of my brothers just can't cope. He cries every time he visits our mother. I call him "Weepy."

ANNETTE, *daughter*

I got fed up with my brother, who never had time to help and didn't think Mom was that much of a problem. So one Saturday I simply took Mom over to his house and left her for the day. He learned a lot.

Daughter

My brother didn't get involved until I went to his office one day and cried. But he just *assumed* because I didn't ask for help. I kept assuming he would come in, but he stayed away because I was capably handling it. But when I did ask him he was right there. So that was a surprise—there were about thirteen years there I wasn't real happy with him.

MARGIE, *daughter*

One of our kids never calls. That hurts a lot.

Husband

The siblings who have a problem going to see my mother, I just sort of came to a conclusion on my own—just leave them alone. Don't try and force them to go.

BELINDA, *daughter*

My wife's life had become shaped by my father's disease. It had become shaped by my detachment from it, and by my mother's furious denial . . .

Margaret and I were living together in different realities. She was inside my father's disease, and I was outside it.

CHARLES PIERCE, *son*

My daughter is 20, and my wife has just been diagnosed with Alzheimer's. They've been at odds anyway, but it's awfully hard to tell a twenty-year-old that she shouldn't argue with her mother any more.

Husband

Mom, I don't think he's having a bad day—I think he's just being an asshole.

SON, *age fourteen*

The hardest part is having to have a father with a mental disability who tries to take over parental duties even though he can't handle it.

SON, *age sixteen*

I saw my sister ruining herself and her relationships with her daughter and others in the family as she took care of her husband. She insisted on doing it all herself, refused to seek professional or paid help, rejected suggestions from the family—and then complained that we were not supporting her.

Sister-in-law

I felt so useless and afraid, as I learned from afar about my cousin's struggle with Alzheimer's, and so guilty that I didn't know how to help.

JENNEKE, *cousin*

❀

Every once in a while, Jenneke would send me an envelope full of especially funny cartoons or clips from the paper. They made me laugh and told me she was thinking of us.

My immediate family "got it" and were very supportive. But two members of my dad's family tried to convince us that it wasn't Alzheimer's, the doctors were wrong, and so forth.

MARSHA, *daughter*

I was never crazy about my sister-in-law, but she was really good through all this, so now I like her a lot.

JUNE, *daughter*

My young grandson doesn't understand why his grandmother loves him one minute and fusses the next. How can I convince him it's not her fault, it's the disease?

HARRY FUGET, *husband*

A few years ago, my son Abraham told me how much he used to hate Sundays. Sundays were when we'd all go out to see my parents. On the way out, my wife and I would always fight, and sooner or later, it would come around eventually to my father, sitting at the end of the couch, wearing a blue floppy hat and smiling vacantly. Abraham was always hot. He was always tired. He hated this Sunday until Tuesday, and on Thursday, he would begin to hate the next one. Half-a-lifetime of hating Sundays.

CHARLES PIERCE, *son*

My little brother used to try to imitate our grandfather's mumblings. He didn't realize that Pete couldn't talk. He thought Pete was playing with him.

LINDSAY, *granddaughter*

It didn't have any emotional effect on me, because as far back as I can remember my grandfather has had Alzheimer's. So I've just grown to accept it. . . . He still has most characteristics he's probably had all his life: calm, sweet, and caring.

CHRISTOPHER SHANKS, *grandson, age fourteen*

I was young when my grandmother was still alive, but I remember her confusion. Even as a nine-year-old I could appreciate my grandfather's dedication. It gave me a sense of what love can be that I will not forget.

Grandson

I was not old enough to know the old Pete. I don't remember that much about when he could talk well, but it was hard to see him lose almost all verbal ability and memory because the disease was stronger. But I knew him, and that was a blessing.

LINDSAY, *granddaughter*

I was trying not to make demands on Nancy Lee until I really needed her help. She had a demanding job and, at that time, a difficult husband. But someone pointed out to me that others in the family may need to help, to know that they are pitching in too. I took a deep breath and asked if Pete could spend a weekend with her while I went away for a brief respite. She agreed immediately. She and her father had a fine time together. My need for a break had become a gift to them both.

My memory is that I kept asking Betsy how I could help, and she kept saying, "No, thanks." I was relieved when she finally asked, because it meant she was finally willing to admit she needed help and because I could contribute something meaningful. It was a special weekend with Dad.

NANCY PETERSON, *daughter*

Friends

I may not remember the words, but I remember the way they made me feel.

JANMINA, *patient*

It is very difficult to tell people that I have an undiagnosed problem of memory. The immediate reply is always, "You haven't got memory loss! You talk quite coherently and intelligently." And then they extricate themselves. I often blow my top and have lost several friends as a result.

LEWIS LAW, *patient*

When I got the diagnosis, I wanted to dig a hole and never leave the house. Then I told one friend, and after that it was much better.

TERRY, *patient*

One of my oldest friends comes and takes me out for lunch every week or so. It's great to get out of the house; it's even great to get away from my wife for a few hours.

WILLIAM, *patient*

What do I want from you? What I need most is your continued love and support. It's not so much in your words, it's that you still care. That you still recognize that I'm alive.

What I don't want is your sympathy. I still enjoy your company, conversations, a card, a phone call. How about e-mail? I enjoy eating out, or a simple board game. Don't let me beat you because you feel sorry for me. I want to beat you fair and square.

No matter how I change, deep inside of me is still that love for you that will never fade away.

CHIP GERBER, *patient*

Social interaction is a major challenge for us persons with dementia.

We're not quite social "lepers." Not being wrapped up in our own thoughts, we can often tune into others' feelings and be warmly responsive to them. TABS (temporarily able-brained persons) enjoy this. But we must be wary that they don't patronize us.

MORRIS FRIEDELL, *patient*

People around me also are now unsure of their role; when you have a disease you are supposed to either get better (then they can all cheer) or get progressively worse and die (and they can properly give you care and mourn). Everyone is poised for some type of action, and there is nothing to do for them; they are unsure of how to support this leaky boat which will eventually sink but for the moment is caught on a sandbar.

JANMINA, *patient*

A small group of incredible friends found a significant way to support and help my family and me. By contacting a wide network of old and new friends, they raised sufficient funds for me to start going to a day program twice a week.

JOHN DURAND, *patient*

My group on the Internet is my lifeline now. These people really understand and are so damned honest about what is going on, and we all continue to keep a sense of humor about our disease.

ALICE YOUNG, *patient*

My friends don't have a clue what it's like. Not a clue.

EVE, *wife*

One weekend my husband and I went to visit Betsy and her husband, Pete, who had Alzheimer's. The first day, Pete and Jim spent about an hour together, chopping up logs for firewood and having a wonderful time working together. On the second day, the subject of firewood came up again. Pete turned to Jim and said eagerly, "Do you like to chop wood?"

I had thought I understood the concept of memory loss before that day. But seeing it in action was different. That happy hour the day before simply did not exist for Pete. For him it had never occurred.

LOIS, *friend*

In the early stages it's hard to get friends to accept what's happening, especially since they seldom see the worst of it. The hardest part is when people say things like, "He seems like the old John," or "You wouldn't believe the things I forget sometimes." They are trying to normalize his symptoms, which are NOT normal. But they could help us live a more normal life—taking him to a movie, keeping us company.

PEGGI, *wife*

People ask, "How is he?" I want someone to ask, "How are *you?*"

EVE, *wife*

I regret not calling on friends sooner for their help. I was loath to accept help from others. It was foreign to my nature. But my reserve contributed to many friends drifting away out of a sense of helplessness. Had I asked sooner, I not only would have eased our burdens, but I might also have retained more friendships.

DANIEL, *husband*

Family and friends treated us like lepers. I understand now that part of it was fear, not wanting to be reminded that they too were eligible candidates for this dreaded disease. I understand, but I will not forgive them. I have not come that far.

NINA P., *wife*

I was shocked when two of my Dad's friends told me—months later—about the day they began to recognize Dad's problems. They saw memory lapses at a meeting and were dismayed when he had no idea where he had parked the car. They worried whether he could make it safely back to Boston. But why didn't they tell me at the time?

Tom, *son*

Two friends came regularly to take Felicity for walks. They didn't come often enough to give me much practical respite, but their regularity gave me psychological respite, the feeling that I was not alone with the disease.

Daniel, *husband*

❧

I am so grateful to the friends and family who kept on coming. They learned to change their conversational style as Pete's abilities faded and to be comfortable with the interactions he could still enjoy. They could learn, as I did, to speak more slowly, to stick to one subject at a time, and to avoid interruptions and direct questions. Eventually, Pete lost the ability to participate in words, but he seemed content to be included with smiles and gestures. And how I needed them to keep me company, at all stages! Pride, if nothing else, helped me to control my irritability when someone else was around.

Invisible Disability

At first, many would tell me that I looked just fine. They could not see my disease. I would wonder what they thought I should look like, what I should be acting like?

CHIP GERBER, patient

I still look the same, and for the most part I can engage in conversations and still maintain my social skills—there is no outward, visible sign at this early stage of the disease that my brain cells are dying and in their death taking away my memories, the essence of myself. . . .

And so, in sharing with family, friends, associates of your newfound loss, rather than a comfort and understanding shoulder to lean on, you find indifference, almost a challenge, to prove your diagnosis—Why on earth would anybody ever choose Alzheimer's??!!!!

JANMINA, patient

Why do people say, "I do that all the time" when we forget the date or can't find a word? If we were diagnosed with malignant melanoma would we hear, "Yeah, I've got freckles all over"?

It's as if invisibility is one of the earliest symptoms, and if we mention Alzheimer's, people get that vacant look. They don't, or won't, understand us . . . but maybe we can understand *them*—after all, for many years we *have been* them.

MORRIS FRIEDELL, *patient*

◆　　◆　　◆

And yet to the outside world she doesn't "look" like she has Alzheimer's, nor does she act it. Is able to appear quite social, just don't ask her ANY question to which you expect a proper reply. For reply she will, but it will have nothing to do with the question . . . SIGH . . .

JANMINA, *daughter and patient*

It's the contrast between the outside and the inside that makes it so confusing. Pete is still so charming, and greets us so warmly, and looks so healthy—and so it's a jolt when we can't talk about poetry any more.

PENNY, *friend*

Airline attendants watched in well-guarded bemusement as I crowded with Muriel into the tiny cubicle that houses the in-flight toilet. I knew what they didn't; if she ever got the door shut—unlikely as that might be—she never could have gotten it open again.

ROBERTSON MCQUILKIN, *husband*

❦

Far into his illness, Pete looked so trim and healthy that most people thought he was in his sixties, not his seventies, and many who met him casually never guessed his problems. Some acquaintances at church thought he was simply quiet or shy. Sometimes—for example, going into a waiting room and telling Pete very simply to take off his coat and where to sit down—I could see the disapproval of strangers and almost hear them saying, "Why is that woman talking to that nice man as if he were a five-year-old?"

The Patient's Changing World

I forget what I was looking for . . . Once the idea is lost, everything is lost . . . you have to be satisfied with what comes to you.

C. S. H., *patient*

Words see me coming and they run away.

JOHN, *patient*

In the nitty-gritty, it means that I no longer drive or cook or now even make the menus. All this stepping back robbed me of my "in charge" attitude, but I wouldn't say I'm exactly humble yet.

CATHLEEN MCBRIDE, *patient*

I can't moderate myself as well. Those skills it was hardest to learn—like controlling my temper—are leaving me now.

ANDY, *patient*

It has been very difficult to be protected, rather than be the protector.

BILL ORME-JOHNSON, *patient*

Don't hurry me, don't rush me, I'm going as fast as I can . . . and that isn't very fast. I think if I moved much slower my wife might call the undertaker. At least I'm up out of bed and dressed. The buzzards aren't circling yet.

CHIP GERBER, *patient*

One day I couldn't figure out how to cross the street. I didn't know which light to walk on. Finally someone came along and I followed her. But I was beside myself—and I thought I had accepted the illness.

DAVE HARRIS, *patient*

Life is really rather surreal, at home away from the "real" world, my early stage symptoms can be pretty much ignored. As with watching a child grow you adjust without even realizing it to the daily changes taking place. It is only when I get out within the "real" world that my limitations become very evident. I become fearful in crowds, panicked. At a restaurant, not always, the choices are overwhelming. I may appear to be listening to a conversation, but somehow I blank out after a short time and am unable to comprehend the words.

JAN MINA, patient

Did you ever take a full minute to decide which way a key goes in the hole? Maybe once, but five times a day? Or look in the phone book and not know which letter follows which letter? Try to add three numbers together and get five different answers? Lose or misplace something five times an hour? I clean up the same pile of stuff four or five times before it gets where it's going, and I used to be the best organizer in the world.

JEANNE LEE, patient

I can't figure out how to turn on the TV any more. If my husband goes out and forgets to turn it on, I'm stuck.

Patient

I'm sitting here wanting literally to scream at the noise of the lawn-mower outside my apartment. I used to love live theatre; the lights and sound left me feeling energized and upbeat. Now they leave me feeling overwhelmed and uncomfortable to the point that I sometimes literally want to scream out to make it go away.

DOREEN, *patient*

Today the time flies by with little accomplished on my part, yet I am exhausted. A doctor told me my entire strength is taken up by fighting my disease. I'm sure this is correct. Even when I'm sleeping it seems I am fighting.

CHIP GERBER, *patient*

I walk through my house where I have lived for over twenty-five years, and I have the feeling sometimes I am in a motel, an unfamiliar place of transition.

THOMAS DEBAGGIO, *patient*

These visual illusions slowly became a part of my life. One was a black caterpillar the size of one of my cats climbing up the white wall next to my closet. . . . Another, I saw a deer under one of the tables at the library. (I had a slight pang of disappointment when I realized it wasn't real. I would have been quite happy to actually meet a deer in the library.)

What should be clear to anyone reading this is that I am having hallucinations. I just call them visual illusions because so far the analytical portion of my brain has always kicked in within a few seconds to let me know what I am seeing isn't reality. I like to think they won't be hallucinations until I lose my awareness that they aren't real.

DOREEN, patient

I stopped driving after I got lost in a neighborhood very near my own. Several times, someone would tell me where to go, and I took notes, but my brain didn't take it in. I had to call the police for help. They were so kind that I felt rather good about the experience. But that was the end of my driving, nevertheless. The risk of possibly hurting someone was too painful.

JIM ANTHONY, patient

Loneliness

This is a very lonely disease.

MARY LOCKHART, *patient*

It's not lonely, in so far as I have Jean and the family and the dogs
. . . it's lonely because I haven't got Me.

BRIAN MCNAUGHTON, *patient*

We've never tried to hide that I have Alzheimer's. But everyone
acts like they don't want to get near because they might catch it.
They don't know how to deal with it. I was always so social before,
but now I don't like to be around people.

BEA, *patient*

If I had a broken leg, I could say, "Hey, I broke my leg, let's talk about it." And you'd tell me about your broken leg, and we'd have a good laugh. But since it's Alzheimer's . . . the stigma is incredible.

People don't know how to approach you. It's like there's a glass barrier between you.

RUTH HARRIS, *patient*

I have been struggling to be contented here while I feel so isolated much of the time and do not have the friends I had up in Minnesota. The children are trying so hard, and I know it is difficult for them, too.

ALICE YOUNG, *patient*

◆　　◆　　◆

The hardest part for a caregiver is the quiet. It kills you.

DON BLISS, *husband*

The word "we" may no longer describe your life.

HARRIET HODGSON, *daughter*

Certainly you find out who your real friends are. The vast majority who haven't had firsthand experience just aren't capable of the empathy. Even if you want to explain what it's really like, they don't want to hear it.

IRENE, wife

"Chocolate," I offered. He stared off into space. I felt so often like I was talking to myself. It was a strange phenomenon, to be so close to someone else and still be alone.

DAPHNE SIMPKINS, daughter

If I just had somebody of my own age group to talk to . . . I mean, I don't think that you are violating any of your vows, having somebody you can talk to. I wouldn't mind having another female, quite honestly, to talk to. Go out and have a beer together.

BRAD, husband

Some of my wife's friends were upset when I started seeing another woman after Julia went to the nursing home, but I was so damn lonely. I had missed going to concerts and parties for several years. I needed the social life. That relationship didn't last. I've done some dating since, but it never goes very far. These new friendships don't hold a candle to the wonderful relationship Julia and I had developed over so many years.

Husband

There were many problems with my husband's illness, but one of the biggest was one I couldn't talk about—he lost interest in sex. I ended up having an affair that ruined several friendships and made me even lonelier. I am thankful I was not more self-destructive during this period.

Wife

I've had a different problem. My husband wants sex frequently— but not much happens when we get into bed.

Wife

At least you had those problems privately. I'm living with my husband's "socially inappropriate" behavior—what a euphemism! I scarcely dare go out with him. He's lost his inhibitions, and I never know when he is going to express sexual interest in a way that frightens others and embarrasses us all.

Wife

I've taken up swing-dancing. It's a lot of fun and I don't need a date.

RICHARD, *husband*

❦

Our dinners got quieter and quieter as Pete gradually lost the ability to report his own doings and had trouble following my anecdotes of the day. It helped, however, when a friend spoke of eating in silence at a religious retreat. After that, sometimes, the meal became a meditation and a time to count all the blessings we still had.

Support Groups

I thought the group would be morose, depressed, and resentful. But we laugh a lot here. It's been a lifesaver.

LEWIS LAW, *patient*

I have to go back to find out who I am and what I am, but here we learn to live with it.

JACOB, *patient*

We indulge in raucous laughter; we also try to practice truth-telling. And a miracle occurs. We leave the group empowered, lifted, and ready to fight the good fight, not against an enemy we can see, but against the power of depression and catastrophic loss.

JIM ANTHONY, *patient*

The group is a safe spot on my life. I can talk freely about anything. And it is extremely gratifying that even though we have memory disorders, we can be a crutch, a listener, an advice-giver, and a friend to others.

BILL ORME-JOHNSON, *patient*

It is such a privilege to be able to connect with someone who is experiencing the same journey as you. Someone who knows the ups and downs, the challenges as well as the joys.

CHIP GERBER, *patient*

The support from the Alzheimer's Association has been absolutely priceless. I didn't feel like I was struggling alone.

MARILYN, *patient*

Many of us do not have the support we need in our own communities, but we do have access to the Internet. The reason the people in my Internet group are doing so well is because we make an effort to help ourselves, but we're helping ourselves by helping other people.

LYNN JACKSON, *patient*

Support Groups

The dementia chat room on the Internet has been such a lifesaver for me. We are all in early onset, and we cope, sharing our stories, experiences with doctors, information, new drugs, etc., and laugh a lot! It is like family to me. Very bright, knowledgeable people.

ALICE YOUNG, *patient*

On with life
On with life
Fight, fight, fight your disease!
It won't beat us
It won't defeat us
It won't bring us
To our knees.

FIGHT SONG OF THE EARLY-ONSET PATIENT SUPPORT GROUP,
BOSTON, MASSACHUSETTS, TO THE TUNE OF "ON, WISCONSIN"

* * *

When I was leaving the house one day, my mother said to me, "Are you going to that family support group you went to last week? You've been a much nicer person since you joined it."

C. K., *daughter*

71

When my mother was first diagnosed, there was so much information I couldn't absorb it or sort it out. But the group has such a wealth of experience; it's a big help.

CLAUDIA, *daughter*

I don't think it's ever too early to go to support group.

MARY, *wife*

In the beginning I found the support group scary—they were describing problems I wasn't ready to hear about, so I stopped going. But it meant a lot to know they were there.

LIZZIE, *daughter*

It's impossible for friends to guess what you are going through. There are things I would never tell anyone who knows my husband—that he had gone weeks without a bath and sometimes peed into the wastebasket. In the support group I learned he was not the only dementia patient to do so—and we could laugh about it! It was such a help to know I wasn't the only one with an unwashed spouse.

Wife

I had to have surgery for an early-stage, very treatable cancer. I told my support group but I didn't want to tell my friends. I couldn't cope with any more sympathy.

DOROTHY, *wife*

The best thing was meeting other kids who had a parent with dementia. We got into a contest about who had the most embarrassing father.

Teenage daughter

Support group didn't work for me. The others were saints.

LIZ, *wife*

I never wanted to join a support group. My problems are mine, and I don't want to listen to somebody else's.

JILL, *wife*

Even a great support group can't do it all. I wanted to rage and weep, but most of the others were being such good sports, trying to make the best of bad luck. That's a better long-term strategy, but I wasn't there yet. It helped me to meet privately with a therapist.

BETH, *wife*

I couldn't stand the support group—the others were too needy. I'd rather take a walk. But I did find a wonderful social worker at the Alzheimer's Association, and our sons and our friends provide a lot of support.

KIT, *wife*

Sometimes I go when I really don't feel like going. I know I get something out of each meeting, and that gets me there.

MARY, *wife*

There were times I didn't go because I couldn't take any more Alzheimer's. But for the most part, support group was the most powerful tool. It offered something no one else could—people who understood what I was living with.

SALLY CALLAHAN, *daughter*

That is why support groups are so valuable. We need a place where we can let go and express our feelings without guilt . . . We need to be able to feel sorry for ourselves and not think we are selfish. Most of all we need to be understood . . . To have people hear us and not tell us we should not think the way we do or feel the way we do is healing.

DOUG MANNING, *author*

This is the most important group in my life—it's my touchstone of what it means to be a human being. We learn about going through hard times and being human.

BETTY, *wife*

It's been lovely, but I have to go scream now.

Anonymous

❦

I'd often go to support group full of woe, feeling very sorry for myself. And most of the time I would end up in awe at the way others coped with problems I didn't have—financial, behavioral, long-standing family issues made worse by the illness. But I also slowly learned not to minimize my own sorrows. Others might have tougher problems, but these sorrows were mine. They were painful in their own right and needed to be grieved.

Money Worries, Legal Tasks

Although I was only fifty-five, I was able to get disability through Social Security. Once that was approved, I was still without income for another seven months before the benefits started. My wife was working, but the only way she could pay the bills was with help from our church.

JOHN DURAND, *patient*

Please, let's get going on the long-term planning while I can still participate. You may have to repeat things a lot, but I deserve to be a part of this process, and I want to make things simpler for you when you'll have to manage without me. Also, we need to talk now about end-of-life issues. I don't want any special measures to keep me alive if I can no longer enjoy my family.

Patient, early stage

◆   ◆   ◆

The disease is bad enough—but now I have to cope with all this legal and financial planning as well. It's hard, and it's even harder to get up the energy to do it.

OWEN, *husband*

Luckily, my wife and I had always had powers-of-attorney for each other, so we didn't have a struggle over that. But she had been the one to manage the household accounts, and my taking over the checkbook was tough. She didn't see why I was so upset that she forgot to record a $5,000 withdrawal.

FRED, *husband*

I had guardianships for both my parents. In Florida, I found that working with the guardianship judge, attorneys, and care manager was much more difficult emotionally and financially than my parents' Alzheimer's. When they moved to Massachusetts, I found the helping system was such a support that it was healing for me as well as useful for my parents. The way this larger system works can either make the stress unbearable or help relieve it.

MARSHA, *daughter*

What I would really appreciate most of all is the chance to get away by myself for a few days. But my husband needs professional care because of other medical problems, and that's $200–300 a day. I can't afford that.

RIFKA, *wife*

Long-term care insurance sounds great—but you can't get it if you've already got a diagnosis of cognitive decline. You can be sure I'm getting it for myself!

Husband

We discovered that my brother had fallen prey to telephone scams and lost thousands of dollars. I think he just said yes to anyone who pitched an investment.

CAROL, *sister*

The biggest mistake we made was going to an attorney who was not an elder law specialist. The regulations are complicated and keep changing. He just wasn't on top of the issues. We found out—too late—that his mistake delayed my wife's eligibility for Medicaid and cost us thousands of dollars.

Husband

Margaret drifted from anger to despair. She'd managed to bludgeon my mother and me into seeing a lawyer to discuss how to protect my father's assets when the time came to find him the nursing home into which my mother had promised she would never put him. Margaret watched as my mother confounded the lawyer, who was under the mistaken impression that we'd all come to her with the same purpose in mind—or, at least that we'd all come to her in fundamental agreement as to how grave the situation really was. Silly lawyer. The smallest thing was a struggle. Margaret would argue that we should do it. My mother would look for the tiniest loophole to avoid doing it. I would try to please both of them and succeed only in further distancing myself from what needed to be done.

CHARLES PIERCE, *son*

It's the money that keeps me awake at night. My husband and I had a good retirement fund—but will it last? He's already been in a nursing home, at $75,000 a year, for more than three years.

DOROTHY, *wife*

❦

I felt abandoned when I learned that the major costs of Alzheimer's weren't covered by our health insurance or Medicare. First, we needed somebody to keep Pete company at home, then a day program, and then assisted living. I had always assumed that our excellent health insurance and Medicare would cover any major medical expenses. But the insurance companies and Medicare classify these types of care as "unskilled" or "custodial." No matter that it's demanding work that is done well only with good training and skill and is best performed in a setting dedicated to dementia care: it is given by staff who do not have nursing degrees. And it is expensive. A good day care program may be $400 a week; assisted living more than $50,000 a year. The best Alzheimer's units in nursing homes in the Boston area now cost $80,000 a year.

Choices

Concentrate on what you have, not what you have not.

Patient

Some with Alzheimer's choose to keep in the closet and that's sad. I find doing the opposite helps me. It helps me handle life in a way to bring hope.

CHIP GERBER, *patient, advocate*

I've always been a fighter, and I sure as hell am not giving up now.

BERNIE REISMAN, *patient*

As long as you are aware of what you can do and can't do, that's okay. Once you accept it, you can decide, "I am going to make the best of this horrible situation," because it is part of your life.

MARGIE SLYNE, *patient*

Knowledge is power, so know about the different medications. With these medications, we are staying better for longer than expected.

LYNN JACKSON, *patient*

Disease is part of the human condition. To see it as evil is to abdicate our strength to overcome, to adapt, to make the best of any situation.

ARLENE BODGE, *patient*

Depression is my worst enemy, usually triggered by messing up something I'm doing—carpentry, fixing a problem in the house, trying to do things I thought were "built in" because I did them so often. One salvation is to avoid such activities and a second is to avoid idle time.

LEWIS LAW, *patient*

You bet I want to participate in those research projects. If I have to have this damned disease, at least we can help others learn more about it.

PETE, *patient*

Choices

I intend to live and grow with whatever the rest of my life brings.

JOHN DURAND, *patient*

Live the moment. Enjoy each day. I even found a word for it. I focus on the "happifying" events of my life—grandchildren, music, and nature.

ELLEN, *patient*

My wife discovered two empty eggshells in the egg carton. My immediate defensive answer was "I didn't do it." But, it seems I did.

We have two choices at this time. We can get all hot and bothered, bent all out of shape, or we can have a good laugh. I choose the latter. Love to laugh even at myself. Makes me feel, oh, so much better than condemning myself.

CHIP GERBER, *patient*

At some point I'm not going to know where the bathroom is. But it may happen tomorrow, or it may happen ten years from now. Why ruin today thinking about tomorrow?

BEN STEVENS, *patient*

I got myself into the darkest hole and tried to commit suicide. But after that I took charge and decided to get well emotionally. Since then, these have been the best two years of my life! I've had a wonderful time and I wake with joy every morning. There is life after diagnosis.

DAVE HARRIS, *patient*

. . .

I see myself daily making choices between wisdom and despair.

LELA SHANKS, *wife*

After reading *The Thirty-Six Hour Day* and so many terrible stories, I thought, "We are going to create our own path." I don't want to read negative things any more.

GEORGIA, *wife*

My first husband also had a long illness and had needed my care. By the time he died, I had lost touch with most of my friends and become very isolated. I'm not going to make that mistake again.

HENRIETTA, *wife*

Choices

My family and I started the Memory Ride, which has raised several hundred thousand dollars for research. We put a lot of work into it. It is one way I do something against Alzheimer's. I do it so that I am not always a victim.

> ERYC NOONAN, *whose family suffers a*
> *rare familial form of Alzheimer's*

The point is, Alzheimer's is a long illness. You can't spend five or ten or twenty years just wringing your hands. My motto is "Alzheimer's with attitude"—or sometimes, "Damn the dementia."

> FRED, *husband*

I finally stopped taking my mother-in-law out of the nursing home for family dinners. She was difficult before she got Alzheimer's and became really nasty as the illness progressed. Her visits were doing too much damage to the rest of us.

> SASHA, *daughter-in-law*

Most important to me has been the discovery that, for us at least, coping is a choice. Dementia is devastating—but it can be managed.

Different people will choose different paths based on their own situation, who they are, where they have been, what they can learn, and what they can handle. No one person can handle dementia care alone. Let me repeat: *You cannot do Alzheimer's alone; don't even try.*

PAM KUNKEMUELLER, *wife*

❦

One of the first newsletters I got from our local chapter of the Alzheimer's Association had a big headline, "Take Control." Give me a break, I thought. This disease is in charge no matter what we do. But eventually I came to appreciate how many choices we do have, and how much those choices shape our experience of the disease. We can learn a lot from the old hands, if we choose to listen, or we can try to do it all ourselves and lose a lot of time and energy in the process. We can choose whether to plan ahead or to let fate overtake us unprepared. We must each choose our own course, but it makes a lot of sense to look at a map first.

The metaphor that works for me comes from river rafting. We can't change the river's relentless downhill course or its variable speed, or remove the dangerous passages of white water. But patients and caregivers can learn to "ride the river": to learn the skills and strategies that minimize the risks, to use but not overestimate our strengths, and to cherish the stretches of calm water.

Denial

Denial works for a while, but it takes too much energy to keep denying. You need the energy to adjust.

Patient

I am astounded at how I go in and out of denial in terms of my disease. I so much want to feel that it will get better rather than worse, and even though I try very hard to stay afloat, lately, I have been feeling that I have a very soggy lifejacket and it will not hold me up much longer.

ALICE YOUNG, *patient*

A degree of denial is essential. Like somebody sipping hot coffee, we sip the truth of our condition carefully and gently.

JIM ANTHONY, *patient*

◆   ◆   ◆

She's in denial. She thinks the only thing that's wrong with her is me. If she could get rid of me, she'd be in perfect shape. She could find everything if I didn't hide it.

HARRY FUGET, *husband*

My stepmother was in such denial of my father's illness. It was frustrating and worrisome. For example, she left the car keys in plain view, and Dad got up in the middle of one night and drove away. The police found him hours later, a few blocks away, with no idea where he was. Even worse, she didn't hide his gun. One day, when he was cleaning it, it went off indoors. Thank God no one was hurt.

LORETTA, *daughter*

Got a call early this morning from my stepdad, he was crying, said Mom had put the tea kettle on, when he told her not to, and burned the stove. She is getting progressively worse, and as much as I try to explain, his words infuriate me. He continues to berate and holler at her, to "shake her up, make her think!" and no matter how hard I try to explain that this is only making matters worse, he chooses not to hear. He is livid that she can still remember how to pour a soda for them both but is clueless to fix a sandwich—yes, I calmly explain, this is normal in an Alzheimer's person. "NO! She is just being stubborn!"

JANMINA, daughter and patient

I knew what was going to happen. We were going to pretend now. We were going to pretend that nothing was wrong, that my father didn't go to the flower store and end up in Vermont. We were going to pretend that he could still order his own food. We were going to pretend that he didn't chase his dead mother down a motel corridor. I felt the truth bending inside me, turning the last three mad days into some familiar shape, and I realized that what I was feeling was the comfort of denial.

CHARLES PIERCE, son

Acceptance is such a slow, irregular process. Eventually I thought I had, at long last, fully accepted the reality of Pete's illness. But again and again I would get these little jolts of recognizing smaller denials. They came in many

flavors—an unrealistic expectation, a blindness to a specific problem, a resistance to suggested help. I would expect him to sit with the suitcase while I went to the ticket counter, and then find him standing behind me—without the suitcase. I bristled when our doctor told me he should stop driving. I would plan something too complicated and recognize ruefully that I'd made the same damned mistake. Again.

Muddling Through the Middle Stage

Many patients and families experience a long middle stretch. We've passed through the initial shock and adjusted in many ways. Although every day is unpredictable, the changes in the disease and in our lives tend to occur gradually, not suddenly. It's not unusual for patients to reach a plateau and go for months or years with little change in symptoms

❦

I think I've lost myself somewhere.

NORMAN, *patient*

I try to read, but it's very difficult. It takes so long to find the next line that I have forgotten what was on the previous line.

BILL, *patient*

I'm forgetting my stories. From now on, you have to tell me my memories.

> SIDNEY, *patient, to his daughter*

When I get frustrated working at something, I put it aside. I say to myself, "Today's not the day."

> *Patient*

I function so well on the computer because I am here in my quiet apartment all alone with just myself and my two cats.

> DOREEN, *patient*

It's not like forgetting. It's not like Alzheimer's patients forget. It's EMPTY.

You know, after a busy day you go home, sit down with a cup of tea and still your mind races, "Did I do this, do I need to do that?" You know, that's normal. I can go and sit and not have a thought for maybe ten, fifteen seconds where there is a blank. But then there is an emptiness that goes with it.

> FRAN NOONAN POWERS, *patient*

I am quite well. I have lost my mental faculties but am perfectly well.

RALPH WALDO EMERSON, *patient, author*

Remarkably, a number of us with Alzheimer's are chipper about it. I'm not sure just why. My guess is that having gotten the heavy news, we decide that we will make the most of being with friends and family and of doing things we love to do. It is a prescription that people without Alzheimer's might try.

JIM ANTHONY, *patient*

It's all about hope. Hope that you never lose your sense of humor.

HERB FARR, *patient*

I'm looking at the long run. We have a long good-bye with this disease. I have time to tell my wife how much I love her.

CHIP GERBER, *patient*

◆　　◆　　◆

It's important to me to know my mother as she is *now*. I need to spend time with her.

LAURIE, *daughter*

While I wept over each loss my husband experienced—resigning from his job, losing his driver's license, fumbling with words—he declared himself a "free and simple man." We hiked, listened to Mozart, savored chocolate.

ANN DAVIDSON, *wife*

On one of these walks, my father climbed into a neighbor's Cadillac and refused to get out, announcing to Margaret that he'd found her a new car.

CHARLES PIERCE, *son*

Muriel, such a self-starting, free-spirited, nonstop doer, became fearful and agitated the moment I left home, felt trapped when she wasn't free to follow me, and "escaped" daily. Many times a day!

ROBERTSON MCQUILKIN, *husband*

Last week my husband told me I looked a lot like his wife—and asked how many kids I had before I died. This week he said he couldn't be married to two people. Sometimes I'm Dot the girlfriend and sometimes Dottie the wife.

DOTTIE, *wife*

When my wife kept asking to go home—and we *were* at home—I would often take her for a ride in the car, and usually she'd be fine when we got home again.

SEAN, husband

He leaves the water running, the stove on at times, lights on everywhere, etc. . . . I check and recheck as much as I can on most things lately but even so many of our affairs are in a state of confusion and what is really hardest is his resentment of my intrusion—"stay out of my affairs!!!" He does not accept or realize my *wanting* to be *helpful* and that is the hardest thing of all for me.

IRENE FRANZEN, wife

My friend's latest bulletins on Mom's dotty doings are always good for a laugh. Because you have to laugh. That's the really, really important thing—you absolutely have to laugh. The crying requires no effort at all. You're going to cry—it's the laughing you have to work at.

MOLLY IVINS, daughter

You can't take care of the person you love unless you take care of yourself. So what have you done for yourself lately?

MAUREEN TARDELLI, *leader of caregiver support group*

❧

Maureen often asked us this question, and it was usually shocking how few of us could answer positively. But there were some good ideas. Buying flowers every week. Scheduling a regular massage. Singing in a chorale. Taking a day off with friends. Taking twenty minutes a day to listen to a relaxation tape. Inviting friends over and cooking a really nice meal. Working out—the endorphins fight depression. Always planning something to look forward to—you can enjoy the anticipation even if the plan doesn't work out.

Grocery shopping together may once have been fun recreation, but not so fun when she begins to load other people's carts and make off with them, disappearing down an aisle into the vast labyrinth we call a supermarket. I've repented of those years of poking fun at "woman talk" as I diligently inquire of a hostess about recipes and call lady friends to learn what kind of a shampoo works best after a permanent.

ROBERTSON MCQUILKIN, *husband*

My father used to go buy lunch at the same deli around the corner every day. They always gave him extra pickles. When I cleaned out his fridge I would find an enormous collection of pickles.

TOM, *son*

I get to feeling mad at myself for the way I'm treating her, like taking her physically to make her sit down, but I have to get her to respond.

BRAD, *husband*

The holidays are tough. Sometimes you don't notice much change from week to week or even month to month. But when you look back a whole year, you see how much has changed since last Thanksgiving.

ADAM, *son*

Sometimes you just have to admit that this is shitty bad luck—give yourself a pity party.

JUDY, *wife*

I finally talked to my doctor about my own depression. It wasn't easy, and I wasn't sure whether it was serious enough to consider medication, but we decided to give it a try—and now I can giggle again.

PEGGI, *wife*

It got more and more complicated to juggle caregiving, my job, and other family matters, but most of the time we seemed to manage. Then some little thing would happen— the toaster oven broke or I got a cold—and it seemed like the end of the world. We were always so close to the edge of chaos—there was no margin, no room to spare.

One Sunday I drove down to take my mother to church. Five minutes before the service she appeared at the foot of the stairs wearing three blouses, one on top of the other, and it took a long time to persuade her to take two of them off. Undressing my mother was one thing I just couldn't do!

When we arrived at the church, we saw that the preacher was a woman, which distressed my mother. She heaved a couple of sighs as the sermon began and then turned to me and said in loud, clear tones, "She thinks she knows more than Jesus!"

Later at lunch she was worried and regretful. At one point she said, "You know, they'll never let us back in that church again."

CARL, *son*

My sister was one of my closest friends. We could discuss anything. And now she's gone, but she's not gone. It was like she decided she didn't want to be my friend anymore, and I couldn't understand why. Even though I fully understand that the disease is the cause, emotionally it's different—it's like she's giving me the silent treatment. When people say to me, "Remember that it's the disease," it infuriates me. Because I do know it's the disease, and I find myself falling short continuously, thank you very much.

JULIE NOONAN LAWSON, *sister and daughter*

At least we know we are dealing with real problems.

BETTY, *wife*

❦

One of the things they don't tell you is that Alzheimer's does a job on the family's memories too. I went through a long phase when I could not bear to look at old photographs: it made the losses too visible. Eventually I got over that, thank goodness, because looking at an album of family pictures became one of the best ways we spent time with my husband. But those old memories were fogged over by years of living with a very different reality.

New Behaviors

It's 5:02 A.M. I'm fully dressed in living room in Boston. Why am I not in bed? The bed is fully made, neat. Pajamas hung up in closet.

6:44 P.M. That is the note I wrote to myself before going to bed, undressed and in pajamas. I thought it was 5:02 *A.M.*, but it was 5:02 *P.M.* Betsy has just come in, found me in bed, asleep, but I woke up easily and looked forward to a cocktail and dinner.

PETE, *patient*

I hate even thinking about my rages . . . but I should talk about them, and the fact that even though I will start screaming when I am in a rage, I feel no anger whatsoever during the whole process.

I don't do well when a lot of people are around, and all the commotion in the airport is the kind of thing that would set off one of my rages. And I hate those things. They make me feel bad afterward and, of course, make those around me uncomfortable when it happens.

DOREEN, *patient*

When I have little control over my emotions, it doesn't mean I'm out of control. When I'm confused and belligerent, I want someone to help me.

JOHN DURAND, *patient*

OK, now this one is fun . . . which is probably a sign of my disease, but I get a kick out of how many things I could care less about now.

If I need to go out to take the garbage out and I'm in my PJs then that's what I'm going out in. It's almost impossible for me to feel any type of embarrassment at anything anymore so I can see no reason at all to get dressed to go take the garbage out. I mean I'm wearing enough clothes not to be arrested for indecent exposure, and since I experience no embarrassment (which is what would keep most people from doing it) at being seen in my PJs, why bother to change?

DOREEN, *patient*

I knew I was in a "funk" and became obsessed with doing things my way and was not being sensitive to other people, particularly not to Linda, my caretaker. When I realized I was way off base, I went downstairs and made amends to her for my mean spirit and not being willing to negotiate. I am very scared for what I may turn into and pray it will not be that way.

ALICE YOUNG, *patient*

❖   ❖   ❖

She follows me all over the house. Follows me around like a puppy dog.

BRAD, *husband*

Jacob has been a "wanderer," taking off by himself. The local police have come to know him and have been very helpful. One time they called and asked me if I knew where my husband was—in the neighboring town in a bridal shop with our big, aggressive German shepherd!

RIFKA, *wife*

I'll never forget the moment when I watched the woman I knew as my mother vanish before my eyes. She was in the hospital for an unrelated illness. Mom didn't like tea, and a hospital orderly had served it instead of the coffee she had requested. She picked up the cup and angrily threw it across the room. It was shocking. I had no idea who this woman was.

SHELLEY FABARES, *daughter, actress*

I nearly died laughing when I overheard a staff member tell the van driver that my sister was at risk of "elopement." I had a vision of her tottering down a ladder to meet her lover . . . but it turns out "elopement" is the term professionals use when a patient takes off on her own when your back is turned.

KEVIN, *brother*

It's the repetitive questioning that drives me up the wall. Every car trip with Dad, he asks again and again, "Where are we going?" I have to play games to keep cool. For a few rounds I explain pleasantly that we are going to visit his cousins in Vermont and chat about the visit. I amuse myself by finding different ways to answer the question. My answers get shorter and shorter. Eventually I time the interval between questions: how long can he go between questions this time? Finally I get smart and put on his favorite tape, "South Pacific," and the music rescues us both.

TOM, *son*

Let's try some new vocabulary here, some reframing. Instead of wandering, how about sightseeing? For incontinence, unplanned leakage. Aggressive—lets her needs be known. Rummaging—good bargain basement technique. Agitated—spirited. Hoarding—a collection of favorite things. For dementia—no worries for tomorrow.

JOANNE KOENIG COSTE, *wife, support group leader*

❧

Pete had never paid any attention to jigsaw puzzles, but one day I picked up a puzzle with a dozen or so big pieces. It had become almost a mantra to say to myself, "It's worth a try." To my surprise, he became completely absorbed. Puzzles became a wonderful way of engaging him and freeing my attention for other tasks. As time went on, he lost the ability to "read" the visual image, or even to recognize that one red piece probably went next to another red piece. It became a process of trial and error, but he found it just as absorbing.

Pete would also spend hours peacefully arranging pennies into patterns—dozens of pennies, usually in circles, rows of circles all across his desk. Although I welcomed the quiet spells, I found it painful to watch this activity. This was a man whose idea of fun had been to learn Greek so he could read The Odyssey *in the original.*

One day, however, I left him to his pennies and took refuge from all the other things I had to do by spending an hour tending to the plants in the tree pits on our street. As I trimmed off dead leaves and cleaned out the chewing gum wrappers, I realized why it made me feel so peaceful. I was bringing order to this tiny part of our world, and order seemed beyond reach in most of my life. When I understood that arranging pennies must give Pete the same comfort, his pennies began to comfort me too.

Adult Day Programs

I like it here. Nobody laughs at me.

W. N., *patient*

I was apprehensive about going to a day program, but I went, and I'm happy with that decision. I often slept all day; now I stay more active physically, mentally, and emotionally. Being involved and accepted makes anyone feel more positive about themselves; it's no different for people with Alzheimer's.

BILL ORME-JOHNSON, *patient*

The day program gave me the means to keep in touch with people. I am not the kind of person who sat at home doing nothing.

MARGIE SLYNE, *patient*

◆   ◆   ◆

My father was outraged when we suggested a day program, but after a while we persuaded him to "volunteer" at the local senior center. He is so much happier now, going off every day to his "work." He looks forward to seeing his friends and being helpful.

Daughter

My wife didn't want to go to a day program, and for a long time I didn't push her. Then it dawned on me—we didn't let our kids choose whether or not to go to school, and I can no longer let my wife make this choice for herself. She needs the stimulus and socializing, and I need the break.

Husband

One Saturday I was out of town and a friend stayed with my husband. He is mostly nonverbal and was very agitated and somewhat threatening. He gestured to my friend to drive right and left and straight and she did. They ended up at the center for his day program. He loves it there and missed his usual routine. It took my friend some time to convince him that it was not open.

RIFKA, *wife*

I used to feel guilty about the challenges my husband gave the folks at the day care program. Then another caregiver at the support group put me straight—they get paid to take care of him, and they get to go off duty at the end of the day.

Wife

❦

It took me much too long to admit it was time to consider an adult day care program. My first visit with the director was a revelation. Jane was wise and compassionate, as I had hoped someone in that job would be. But I had not guessed how much the professional perspective would help. Jane knew lots of people with Alzheimer's, not just one. She could draw on years of experience to interact with my husband and to deal with problems I was trying to figure out alone. She could rejoice in Pete as he was, instead of always mourning the loss as I did.

Nonetheless, on his first day I was as twitchy as a mother sending her child to school for the first time. I didn't guess, until I tried it, how good it would be for me to know that Pete was busy and happy in safe hands.

Getting More Help

Thank you for baby-sitting me. Here's a dollar.

PATIENT, *to his twelve-year-old grandson*

The caregivers are doing their darndest, and they deserve their time away from us, because it can be very tedious. I can be very tedious, and I'm aware of that.

CARY HENDERSON, *patient*

There are people who very early in this process said you must get someone to do your checkbook. I wasn't at that point yet. It was very insulting to me to be told, "Never mind what you think. This is what I think you should do." There is a lot of that attitude in these well-intentioned people. I fought like hell during every single step in getting help. . . . Then eventually I think, "I really do need it now," and I do it.

JEAN, *patient*

I have trouble getting dressed. So, I don't do it myself anymore.
I have a girl who comes in and does it for me. If she's not here, Joe
can do it, but it's a hassle. I don't know what to do and he doesn't
know what to do, so neither of us does anything. Maybe I should
join a nudist colony!

BEA, *patient*

⁂

I like to help take care of my grandpa. It's fun to spend time with
him, probably 'cause I love him so much.

CHRISTOPHER SHANKS, *grandson, age fourteen*

Thank God for outside help. It's so hard to take the first step—
afterwards you say why didn't I do it sooner.

MARY, *wife*

I would hire someone to come in. She would fire them by the time
I got them, I mean, I would hire, she would fire.

JAN, *daughter*

I found it so hard to learn to ask for help. But when I finally admitted to a need, someone or something usually came forward to help. For example, people from our church would take turns spending an hour with my wife, so I could go out to do errands or just for a walk.

TONY, *husband*

Sometimes a friend would call up and offer some practical help—taking our car to be inspected, coming over to help plant the garden or clean out the basement. What a gift!

PEGGI, *wife*

One thing I've learned is that whatever solution a family develops for someone with Alzheimer's is by definition only temporary. With my mother, we're increasing the hours spent with the aides, but at some point she'll need them all the time or something else.

RUTH MACNAUGHTON, *daughter*

Changing his diapers is not good for me.

Daughter

My husband didn't do well in the day program, so I began to search for people who could help at home. When they came, I began to recognize how exhausted I had been, emotionally and physically, doing it all myself. Even better, we gradually developed into a new little family, all of us caring for Donald, sharing our very different lives.

BETTY, *wife*

I was finally facing the reality that I should no longer leave Pete at home alone for long, but I also knew I needed to refresh myself. I began by hiring my niece Kathy, then in college. She helped me learn that sharing the care was good for all of us. That made it much easier for me to turn to strangers eventually. Even so, each new step seemed huge—placing an ad, getting a college student to come visit, hiring a "housekeeper" whose real job was to keep an eye on Pete and get him lunch.

These people came for a few hours a day, but friends and an Alzheimer's counselor had been urging me to take a longer break, for respite. Finally, I was ready, prompted by my nephew's wedding on the West Coast. The woman who would stay with Pete came to our home a week before the trip. She quietly helped me realize she knew a lot more about caring for someone like Pete than I did. My tension evaporated: we had found the Alzheimer's equivalent of Mary Poppins. Alas, two days later she had a medical emergency and had to cancel.

When I met her substitute, she seemed capable, but she did not calm me in the same way. Only then was I really forced to confront and define my fears. My friends had been happy with every aide sent by this agency. How bad could it be? I imagined various worrisome scenarios. Finally I had to admit that Pete would be as safe with her as with me and probably about as content.

That's the way it turned out. Yes, I worried a lot, and I called home often, but things went well. And the trip and the wedding were great.

Other Medical Matters

I can't imagine getting this diagnosis without getting depressed.
We need to deal with that too, treat the whole person.
Therapy works!

DAVE HARRIS, patient

Depression has become the major problem—everything I do reminds me of my increasing incompetence. It goads me to the attitude, "To hell with it all; why stay alive?" Better medication has helped, but it took considerable time to sort out which medications and what doses were effective. The coloring agent in one drug caused a violent allergic reaction.

LEWIS LAW, patient

I was a good candidate for coronary bypass—but that would have meant being under general anesthesia for eight to ten hours. The neurologists thought it likely that long sedation would add to the memory issues and it was best to be conservative. So in consultation with our doctors we chose a less invasive procedure, cardiac stents.

TERRY, *patient*

You know, I've got Alzheimer's and can never remember what I'm not supposed to eat.

SARGENT SHRIVER, *patient*
(chastised for eating lots of french fries)

♦   ♦   ♦

One of the problems is that a person with Alzheimer's doesn't really know when he is sick. He doesn't remember that he doesn't usually feel this bad.

MAUREEN REAGAN, *daughter*

Felicity was unable to understand her gynecologist's instructions to change into a johnnie. My efforts to remove her clothing were

124

met by her equal resolve to remain clad. Teenage years came flooding back as I attempted to remove her panties, while she adamantly yanked them back up. By the time I finally wrestled Felicity into her johnnie, she was so agitated I could only keep her from getting out of the examining room by putting my arms around her. She understood this embrace as an invitation to dance. She seemed to enjoy our little ballet, while I was exhausted. The doctor returned, mid-twirl, leaving me to wonder if he thought we both had dementia.

DANIEL, *husband*

My sister noticed that Mom was having difficulty holding down any food. She also seemed very weak and despondent. When we questioned her about how she felt, she was "just fine." We took her to the hospital and discovered she'd had a severe heart attack. You need to be suspicious, doubting, persistent, and very observant to diagnose illness in an Alzheimer's patient.

S. G., *daughter*

My mother's wrist was inexplicably swollen, so I took her to see a renowned rheumatologist. She couldn't talk, and by the time she we left that office, three different doctors had pushed and twisted her arm. The theories, expressed without compassion, ranged from a broken bone to a blood clot and pancreatic cancer. I heard the senior member say to the others, "What we are doing here is veterinary medicine."

Mother and I remained remarkably calm during all this. But we were both exhausted by the time she had an ultrasound and an X-ray, and had to struggle down some stairs and back to the car. As I drove her home, I was crying and shaking all the way—and furious. No doctor, no matter how brilliant, should push and prod an old lady and tell us cancer would be the best outcome. I hope when his time comes someone decides he's hopeless and can be treated like an animal.

WYN, *daughter*

After spending one night in a chair in Dad's hospital room, we decided it was well worth the money to hire a sitter. He couldn't be alone: he'd head off to the bathroom without any awareness he was hooked to an IV pole.

TOM, *son*

He has cardiac problems and diabetes. His inability to understand the importance of diet restrictions and his great love for food affects both of them. It's harder for him to take his own blood sugars now—and when he does, the numbers don't mean anything to him anymore.

MARY, *wife*

I didn't know then that aggression and disruptive behavior are often signs of physical discomfort in an Alzheimer's patient. Now that I do, I suspect my father was in pain during these episodes, but that he himself had no understanding of this in a conventional sense and certainly no way to say, "I hurt." Instead he incorporated the pain into his delusional life. "They" were hurting him—badly. "They" needed to be fought off. And when he fought them off, "they" needed to restrain him, to tranquilize him, in order to maintain some kind of order for the sake of the other patients on Level Four.

SUE MILLER, *daughter*

❧

Pete had been losing his appetite for some time and was visibly declining. The staff at his assisted living unit thought it was just the progression of Alzheimer's. I considered taking him to the doctor, but I couldn't see how the visit would produce any useful information. At the last appointment, Pete had refused to take his clothes off. By then he couldn't talk anymore, and the three of us had stared at each other largely in silence. No one suggested a blood test until he began to show a little jaundice. The test led to the discovery that he had gallstones, which were promptly removed. His appetite and cheerfulness returned immediately.

"Childishness" and Dignity

I call this "growing down"—I'm not going to learn again to do things on my own.

BOB, *patient*

This is like growing younger. So many "normal adult" things matter to me very little now or not at all. I look at adult behavior and find it kind of silly sometimes because it's so wrapped up in so many rules, so many rules that when you get right down to it are reinforced by the use of embarrassment if you break them . . . and once you lose the capacity to feel embarrassment, the rules start to appear very silly.

I just heard myself burp loudly. I used to be quite ladylike, but for some strange reason now it makes me chuckle when I hear myself burping loudly. Am guessing that is just more of that part of me that is growing more childlike . . . It *is* definitely a behavior change for me!!!

DOREEN, *patient*

I am more aware of the world now, the tiny insignificant things especially. I am beginning to be more childlike. For an artist this may have some advantages. As a fifty-eight-year-old man it has many drawbacks. I am losing precious memory, and complex ideas become twisted. I am becoming a child again against my will.

THOMAS DEBAGGIO, *patient*

I'm becoming more childlike now. I enjoy the things children enjoy. I don't have the same responsibilities. I can do what I want. I really am a child.

BILL, *patient*

❖   ❖   ❖

One evening I told my roommate that I was going to "baby-sit" my uncle—and then felt terrible. He's not a baby or a child, even though he needs somebody with him.

KATHY, *great-niece*

Some people talk about patients becoming childish again or reverting to childhood. That concept is really misleading—these are mature adults. "Childlike," maybe, but not children.

MAUREEN TARDELLI, *leader of caregiver support group*

❧

I've been brooding over this comment: I both agree and disagree. I hate hearing someone say that a person with dementia is childish, and yet there are many similarities— some of them wonderful. My husband often responded with a direct delight to something I was too busy to notice. There was a poignant phase when Pete, age eighty-one, and our grandson Zachary, age four, enjoyed the same puzzles and toys—and both had trouble taking turns. I could see, too, that my daughter-in-law and I were using the same strategies—speaking simply, trying to prevent overtiredness, providing a diversion to avert distress.

Maureen's point, I think, is to remind us that everyone deserves to be treated with courtesy and dignity.

Both my parents had Alzheimer's, and I don't think they did have mature emotions in the last years—strong feelings, yes, sad or angry or happy, but not what I think of as "mature."

As I helped my parents, with feeding, or walking, or taking them to the bathroom, I often thought how their parents had gone through this years ago, with great joy. Now I have the privilege to do the same thing at the end of the life cycle, closing the circle. I often imagined my grandmothers taking care of them as babies and watching me mother my parents.

MARSHA, *daughter*

It is possible to have a high quality of life and live with dignity while suffering with Alzheimer's. I want to do my best to enable my mother to live the way I want to live in my old age.

RUTH MACNAUGHTON, *daughter*

I see Hughes today as still contributing. His task at this time is to be an Alzheimer's patient. . . . He requires no pity, only respect. . . . It is through the profundity of his humanness that he is training me. I believe he knows somewhere inside that he is still fighting for the human dignity of the individual. Every Alzheimer's patient offers us an extraordinary opportunity to discover more enlightened approaches to patient care and to advance the human race to new frontiers of understanding.

LELA SHANKS, *wife*

It isn't Alzheimer's that takes away the person's dignity; it's other people's reactions that do.

JOANNE KOENIG COSTE, *wife, counselor*

Truth or Comfort?

I have really struggled with the honesty issue. What do you say to someone who thinks she has no money to pay bills and will lose everything she owns if she doesn't get home to a job she retired from years ago? I couldn't find any reason for telling her over and over that she has a horrible degenerating disease.

Sometimes saying nothing was better than anything I could say . . . what she needs is comfort and security—not the truth. The truth won't change anything.

N. B.

My guilt was that I couldn't be up-front. That I couldn't be honest with her and say, "You can never go home."

JENNY, daughter

It's a fiblet—a little lie for a very good reason. The choice is to enter the patient's world and comfort, not to confront.

JOANNE KOENIG COSTE, wife, counselor

I didn't exactly lie to my mother. I just left out all the information that would upset or confuse her.

Daughter

It's not a lie—it's an honorable deception.

Husband

I welcomed the sense of usefulness and purpose my father's delusions gave him. I was glad when he reported he'd done things—familiar Dad-like things—that I knew he hadn't done. I lied. I went along with his mistakes. I still don't know if this was right or wrong, but I would do it again. I would choose to have my father feel happy and competent in some parallel universe, rather than have him build something from Popsicle sticks or learn line dancing.

SUE MILLER, *daughter*

Never attempt to reason with a person who has lost her reason!
JOANNE KOENIG COSTE, *wife, counselor*

Alzheimer's as a Teacher

I used to be so busy trying to make myself loveable. Now, with Alzheimer's, I'm even busier loving others.

Patient

For the first time I have become a very needful recipient of voluntary help. I understand and appreciate much more the incredible efforts that these people put forth. I'm deeply grateful and have learned to accept such help gracefully.

LEWIS LAW, *patient*

I was in a black, black pit, but my wife dragged me out, and I realized I was doing it wrong. Forget about the life back then—there's a lot I can do now.

It's criminal not to enjoy yourself, to do good things with family and friends. I do lots of things I should have done years ago when I was too busy working.

BERNIE SHAPIRO, *patient*

. . .

I have learned, and this lesson was easy, that there cannot be too many hugs and kisses. I say "I love you" often. In addition to being true, it gives assurance and reduces fright.

M. S., *husband*

We talk a lot about learning to live "in the moment." By golly, the Alzheimer's patients know how to do that—and can teach us too.
Staff member in Alzheimer's day program

"Keep it simple, stupid!!" Why is that so hard to learn?

BETH, *wife*

Alzheimer's is a fierce teacher, full of paradox. I have despaired and felt isolated. But Alzheimer's can teach the joy of connecting, however small. It can teach how to find pleasure in fleeting moments, how to find dignity in people no matter how impaired. It can teach that much of a person's essence remains despite dreadful losses.

Alzheimer's has also let me realize my own strength. Much as I love Julian, I've learned to build a meaningful, happy life without him. I stay emotionally connected, while at the same time letting him go.

ANN DAVIDSON, *wife*

There is a world of difference between curing and healing, and healing is by far the more important. Healing is just as possible with dementia as it is with any of life's other challenges.

PAM KUNKEMUELLER, *wife*

This man, my father, continues to teach me about life and about myself. How can I separate how I feel about him "now that he has Alzheimer's disease"? I cannot.

CEDRIC SHANKS, *son*

I'm learning to enter into a new world, my mother's world. If she thinks I'm her mother, that's fine—what joy it gives her to see her mother!

MARSHA, *daughter*

My father, who is the primary caregiver, has really surprised me. He was always the quiet one, a true Yankee. My mother was the social one. But he has become able to talk about his feelings—he even sought out a social worker.

KIT, *daughter*

Confronting this reality head-on caused me to replace my prayer for my father's "cure" with a prayer for his and my mother's happiness, no matter what. Without realizing it, I was beginning to make the facts of my father's illness a part of my reality, and a new relationship with him and my mother could now begin to take shape. . . . Now, when I look into his eyes, I see a man whose life has exemplified courage, integrity, dignity, and wisdom; a man who cared deeply for others and is deeply loved; a happy man, whose life continues to bring joy to others: my father.

SHELA OMELL RICHARDS, *daughter*

I guess we learn flexibility along with renewed patience with this damned disease. We should be almost perfect by the time we're through with it.

JUDY, *wife*

❧

I have learned so much about the power of the human spirit. I have met so many patients and family members struggling against difficulties and despair, day after day, month after month, year after year, and yet, somehow, finding the roses in the desert. I have met staff members who didn't have much education or training but have the gift of calming a patient and bringing a smile. I have met dedicated professionals. Most of all, I learned how much each of us can grow and how much we can help each other. It fills me with awe.

Dark Parts

There is a wide emotional difference between knowing you will die one day in the future and living with the knowledge you have a disease that slowly squeezes the life from you in hundreds of unexpected ways, and you have to watch it happen while those who love you stand by unable to help you.

THOMAS DEBAGGIO, patient

I'm not sure why I cannot be honest with those around me, with the exception of Wade, till I get to the point where I have pushed myself into depression, and feelings of failure, and guilt for the destruction this disease has wrought on Wade. . . .

    These are not new demons—they have come to haunt me before, and each time Wade patiently tries to make me see what is his reality, and how mine has become distorted. The tears are uncontrollable, when finally released—why do I find it so necessary to push myself to these extremes?

JANMINA, patient

+ + +

Because we are not volunteers for this new and difficult job, beginning caregivers often experience a concentrated excess of hostile emotions—from anger to hate to resentment to rage to bitterness to self-pity to embarrassment to fear. We may run the gamut of all our negative feelings in one moment.

LELA SHANKS, *wife*

I was just exhausted all the time. And I just felt real helpless and powerless. Like it was an out-of-control train and it was all I could do to keep it in the tracks. And I felt very—not angry, angry is not really the word, I don't know what the word is. I felt that he was so gypped. You know, my mom and dad had these grand plans for when he retired. I've seen him work like a dog his whole life and not get to enjoy it. They never got to do all of the things they wanted to do together.

IRENE, *daughter*

Quite suddenly I had a breakdown. Shouting and sobbing and screaming. No reason for it. Iris, my wife, at first smiled at me incuriously. She did not seem at all surprised. And not very interested, either. What had happened to me? Why had I suddenly popped off? . . . Abruptly, it seemed, heart had quietly escaped from me. And courage. And will. I could go on doing all the things I had to do, but none of them seemed to help us anymore.

JOHN BAYLEY, *husband*

I had an awful fight with my father, and then I completely broke down, crying, "I want my daddy back, I want my daddy back."

Daughter, age eighteen

I envy those in my support group who talk about their spouse as cooperative, kind, helpful, or loving. My husband used to be those things but is now often angry, combative, mean, crass, or distant. I've even lost the enjoyment of remembering how wonderful he used to be. The personality change was gradual and began long before his actual diagnosis. Now when I try to remember earlier times I am simply overcome with despair about today.

Wife (whose husband has a frontal dementia,
which is more likely to cause personality change)

Everyone else I know who had a terminal disease lived only twelve or eighteen months. Mom just passed the five year mark from diagnosis with dementia. You don't even want to know what I would give to know that her journey would end within the next year or year and a half.

Dale, *daughter*

Well, I'm glad that some people have the experience of finding a newer, deeper relationship with the person they take care of. For me, that's bullshit. It's been nothing but loss and unremitting labor.

Wife

My biggest fear is that I will end up hating my husband.

Maggie, *wife*

No, it's the disease we hate. Hating the disease was one thing my husband and I could do together.

Pam, *wife*

I hate—no, not him, but what's happening to him. Then I feel bad about myself.

Wife

Anger

Has anyone told you about the rage?

Bart, patient

◆ ◆ ◆

Sure I get angry. But I got angry before Jane got sick. I feel it's part of being human. I give myself a certain amount of time to be angry and then I get over it.

Husband

Felicity had a paranoid phase in which she was unremitting in her anger and accusatoriness to me. I frankly and deeply hated her during this time and looked forward to some institution taking her off my hands. Naturally my guilt for having such thoughts was as profound as my rage. I am pleased to report that I have almost entirely forgiven myself for my all-too-human response to a very grueling phase in her illness.

Daniel, husband, a psychiatrist

I was not just exhausted from the extra load of physical work; I was exhausted from feeling angry. . . . Was there an alternative to anger?

I observed that the critical time for me to avoid anger when working with Hughes was in that initial moment when he refused to cooperate (most likely because he did not understand; after all he is demented). I find that when I accept him as he is and "lean into the pain," my anger is mitigated. . . . In those too rare times, Hughes and I work together inseparably for his care.

LELA SHANKS, wife

I have yet to meet an Alzheimer's caregiver who did not feel anger. Some claim they don't, but their body language and choice and delivery of words belie their denial. There are many reasons to feel anger at Alzheimer's—the loss of a loved one in such a bizarre and difficult way, the lack of understanding from others, the myriad problems, and the condescending or brusque treatment from some professional caregivers.

Finally, caregivers often feel anger at their patient and at themselves. It helps to understand the differences between sadness and grief and depression and to find ways to express anger. It helps to identify Alzheimer's as the culprit and the source of the anger, rather than blaming the patient or themselves.

SALLY CALLAHAN, *daughter, support group leader*

❧

I went through a long, tough phase in which I could seldom control irritability and anger at my husband. My mind knew that it was only human to be irritated by hearing the same question again and again and again and that it wasn't his fault, but I would still blow up on the fourth or fifth reply, then hate myself even more. It was one of the most corrosive experiences I have ever had.

But then, by the grace of God, I was helped to understand that my anger came mostly from grief. I had not recognized that I was grieving as well as coping with all the practical challenges. I think I was afraid to face the grief, fearing I would be overwhelmed by it. Instead, things went much better for me and for Pete when I faced the grief and learned to cry. His repeated questions were still irritating, but when I lost my patience, it was just a loss of patience, not a corrosion of the soul.

Grief

But you must mourn. For me it is a private mourning. I take stock of my treasures that are endangered—reading, music, theater. I wonder how this disease will affect my friendships.

JIM ANTHONY, *patient*

I guess when I have lost enough brain cells that I can no longer recognize my friends, I am sure they will believe in my diagnosis, and they will seek solace and comfort for the loss of our friendship, family ties—as I grieve now, alone.

JANMINA, *patient*

After my daughter Becky left, I became very very sad. Took a walk but I still felt depressed. I realize I am grieving my losses of ability to function and it is getting worse. I know I am in the middle stages now, and Becky and I agreed that my time to live a rather independent life is coming to an end.

ALICE YOUNG, *patient*

❦

I went to the bookstore hoping to find something helpful on grief. Instead, the books all talked about "letting go." I could see some wisdom in that, but how can you "let go" of someone whose care occupies most of your mind? How can there be four million American families living with dementia and no books recognizing our kind of grief? I felt even lonelier than before.

Now he's in the final stages. It's grieving continuously, watching someone you love slip slowly, slowly away.

NANCY PETERSON, *daughter*

I think I'm grieving more for myself and for the loss of my life. I'm forty-three years old, and I can't leave my house because I can't leave my mother alone.

MARTHA, *daughter*

I continually say that she has one foot in heaven now, and I wish that God would take the other foot, because it is such a sad situation.

BOB, *husband*

Grief

I never recognized that I felt grief until recently. It was a word used to describe somebody going through a tragic emotional time. Never a word to be associated with me. Now I see that it started the day of diagnosis and it hasn't ended.

MARY, *wife*

You can't process the grief with the person who's dying, and that's what's so hard.

IRENE, *daughter*

One blessing is that I have gotten through a big part of the grief process. I have now accepted the husband I have today. I have learned to go with his flow whenever possible. This is a wonderful gift. It has taken a few years to reach this point, but it has freed me of the need to control every situation. I often feel as if I divorced the former husband and married a similar man. He looks the same but responds very differently to most parts of our former lifestyle.

JANE, *wife*

The grief of Alzheimer's is what I call slow grief. We begin to grieve at the time of the diagnosis but feel we must keep a good front for our loved one and the family. We try to not grieve, or if we do, we try not to let it show. Each step of the disease brings more and more loss and more and more pressure to be positive and not lose control. We grieve in little private spurts. As long as we are the caregivers we can't find the time or the place to let go and grieve. The longer we bury our feelings, the deeper they get and the harder they are to bring up. Gradually we become exhausted and numb. When death comes, it is hard to find the feelings we need to express our pain.

My wish for every caregiver is that you will find some folks who will give you permission to grieve, that they will let you feel, let you cry. I hope you find someone who will understand.

DOUG MANNING, *counselor*

❦

I completely lost my temper with a young social worker who said I was experiencing "anticipatory grief." Antici-patory, hell! There is nothing anticipatory about having dinner with my husband who can no longer carry on a conversation. There is nothing anticipatory about Pete's loss of so many activities and relationships he loved or our loss of things we had enjoyed together. These losses are here and now.

I later learned that "anticipatory grief" can be a technical term, used by professionals only to indicate that the grief takes place before the death. Well, it's a lousy term. It made me feel that my grief was abnormal, and I couldn't believe it was.

Issues for the Soul

What keeps me going? Ultimately, I want to leave behind a message for my descendents that when life pitches them a curve they don't have to curl up and fade away. They can get back on their feet and continue being the persons the Source of Life meant them to be.

MORRIS FRIEDELL, *patient*

The bottom line is—I'm in God's hands . . . and the medical community's. And hopefully they're in God's hands.

BUTCH NOONAN, *patient*

I don't know what I would do if I didn't have my faith. That's the only thing that holds me together.

BEA, *patient*

There are days when I look at myself and I don't like the person I see myself becoming. This is hard because I have spent a lifetime working hard to meet my spiritual goals for this lifetime. And while no human will ever be perfect, I was fairly happy with who I slowly became over time. There was more about me that I liked than that I didn't like. That is slowly reversing as this disease progresses, and I find myself becoming less tolerant of others. I find myself easily becoming frustrated and annoyed and have to work much harder to make sure that I behave in ways that are spiritually appropriate. (Socially appropriate I could care less about anymore, but spiritually appropriate is very important.)

DOREEN, *patient*

The lake has been like glass this evening, with the pine trees reflecting in the water, and the setting sun all oranges and reds reflecting in the water. Then the loons started calling as they greeted the night.

I feel so fortunate to live in a place like this—I cannot bear the thought of getting to the point of not comprehending where I am, and yet somehow I know that my soul will always know and that God will be with me. I feel so calm tonight that I almost feel I do not have this disease—what a lovely feeling!

ALICE YOUNG, *patient*

• • •

Praying doesn't help, and I don't feel like thanking God for my blessings when my loved one suffers with this illness.

Anonymous, from the Anger Wall

Please, God, I'd trade places with her in a minute. Don't do this to her. I can't lose my faith, not now—please carry me now.

Daughter, from the Anger Wall

Here was a woman who had given her life to her family and her belief in her God, and then why did this happen to her? I was in real anger.

JAN, *daughter*

Prayers have become all-compelling as the only means I know for facing crisis after crisis with Hughes and successfully getting through each day.

LELA SHANKS, *wife*

When I prayed at all, I prayed prayers of thanksgiving for the unfathomable power of my wife's compassion.

CHARLES PIERCE, *son*

When my husband, Jim, became agitated at communion time, our priest guessed correctly that he was concerned that he could no longer make a coherent confession. He said, "Jim, you don't need to worry about making your confession anymore. Don't be troubled that you can't find the words. Sin requires an intention and consciousness that you have lost. You are living in a state of grace."

PAM, *wife*

I was angry at God, and I had to work through that. My mother used to say, "If you have a problem, you talk to God." Well, I'm sure that sometimes the way I talked to God wasn't the best, because He and I really had some talks. Why? Why did this happen in our family?

MARGIE, *daughter*

It's about being mad at God. It's about having a loving and supportive family. It's about maybe that's God's way, helping you through *them*.

MARY JESSUP AMONETTE, *wife*

I questioned God a lot, just wondering why it would happen to such a young person as my mother. I spent a lot of time in prayer and I journaled a lot, and I can't say that now I have the answer. I don't.

SUZUKI, *daughter*

I have become a more spiritual person because I know that I get a lot of strength from doing a bit of meditating and just taking time to myself. It's like having my church at home.

CORINNE, *wife*

I have begun to realize that I have to see Alzheimer's as more than saying good-bye. It is discovering the new person that emerges as the old one fades. It is accepting the grace God gives me to keep on loving this new someone despite my anger and grief and sometimes even despair.

That's the key to it all, isn't it? Finding God's grace in the middle of the chaos dementia brings to our lives. Could there be any good in this long good-bye? Only the good of learning to love more perfectly.

LAURI COVINGTON GRANTHAM, *daughter*

His body is covered in urine and excrement, and he can't figure out what to do about it. "Help me, God," I repeat my prayer. I fall to my knees, and in faith that I will last long enough to do the work, my hands go where they do not want to be. I begin stripping my beautiful daddy. It is not an easy job to undress a man who cannot follow directions as well as a child.

Just as I felt my daddy's presence and his need of me before I descended the stairs, I felt the presence of Love Itself—God—in the room while I tended my sick daddy. Strength not my own moved my body. Strength not my own moved my daddy.

DAPHNE SIMPKINS, *daughter*

When it became too difficult to get Jim to church and up to the altar rail, a Eucharistic minister brought communion to us, first to our home and then to the nursing home, week after so many weeks. After a while Jim no longer responded to the readings and prayers. But the moment she offered the Host, it captured his attention. This lifelong ritual sustained him until he could no longer swallow. I will always be grateful to the church, the faith, and the individuals who made our continued membership in that communion possible.

PAM, *wife*

If you believe in the concept of a soul, then you have to believe that the soul doesn't get Alzheimer's any more than it gets cancer. Maybe the soul has an awareness of the life around it that transcends the body or the ability to communicate. . . . Maybe, just maybe, our people have the unique experience of being able to live in two worlds, ours and a freer one that allows them access to insights and awareness we can't even begin to fathom.

BEVERLY BIGTREE MURPHY, *wife*

❦

Alzheimer's has been the making of my soul. For one thing, it sent me back to church, where I began again to confront some of the crucial spiritual issues. I needed that larger context for our sorrows—and our blessings. I needed the stimulus of new friends and a community of faith. And I had been so lucky with most of my life: Pete's illness was far and away the most serious adversity I had encountered. I felt newly connected to others in pain. I was being initiated at last into truths and mysteries I had tried to avoid.

Gifts

People with Alzheimer's have gifts to give. Do not underestimate our strengths and wisdom. We do not survive Alzheimer's without learning a thing or two.

JIM ANTHONY, *patient*

I ask you to treat our words and images as gifts. Gifts given to bring hope in the face of despair, love in the face of indifference and pity, knowledge where there is ignorance, laughter to unite the tears of sadness with the smile of God.

BRIAN MCNAUGHTON, *patient*

I am really only beginning to enjoy the *now* of life, something that completely passed me by before. So, all in all, I would describe Alzheimer's as a new stage in a wonderful life, no less challenging or interesting than all the earlier stages.

CATHLEEN MCBRIDE, *patient*

I find myself more visually sensitive. Everything seems richer: lines, planes, contrast. It is a wonderful compensation.

MORRIS FRIEDELL, *patient*

One of the things that I like about this disease is the fact that it keeps me so much in the present . . . it is as if mindfulness, which is normally a struggle for most humans, is now almost a piece of cake for me. Buddha said the cause of suffering is craving. And it is true that as I find myself with fewer and fewer desires, I am more and more content (most of the time). While I'm not thrilled about the end result of this dementia, most of the time I can put those thoughts aside and dwell just in the present . . . and I see that as a gift of this disease.

DOREEN, *patient*

I would like to mention all the good things that have come to me since I learned I have Alzheimer's. I have found a very warm, supportive partner. My friends have rallied around. I have the time to write poems, stories, letters to friends. I lead a poetry group for elders. I have the time to enjoy good music. My cat tells me every day how much she enjoys having me around. I have time to meditate. I have time to be myself.

JIM ANTHONY, *patient*

◆   ◆   ◆

I believe that my mother's illness brought her gifts as well, as I know it did to Wayne and me. She was our blessing, although a fierce one.

TERRY BALTZ, *daughter*

A true gift from my parents—Alzheimer's taught me to be more patient and more emotionally available than I ever imagined possible.

MARSHA, *daughter*

Dad is much warmer. This disease has given the family the opportunity to work out some relationships.

LEIGH SAUNDERS KITCHER, *daughter*

Something happened that made me feel I really had to have a good talk with my father before it was too late, although I was fearful that he would react in anger. I told him how much I admired him in many ways and also some things that had been very hard for me—especially the way he lost his temper with me and my brother. Dad then tearfully recounted how his own dad had been hard on him in many of the same ways. We both realized how things are passed down through the generations, despite our best intentions. We apologized to each other. What a moment this was—I finally understood Dad's wrath and was freed from the bonds of my childhood. Only much later, as a father of two teenagers, did I get the additional perspective of just how hard it is to deal with teenagers. The fact is, I was pretty volatile fuel for a father's anger.

JOHN PETERSON, *son*

❦

Pete told me about that conversation. He was in awe that he and John had been able to talk about such things and was grateful to John. He told me he had never talked with his own father about anything so important.

Gifts

We learned about the kindness of strangers—most dramatically, the day I got a call from a woman who never even gave her name. She reported simply that my mother had missed her train and would be on the next one. (We learned later that the person who drove Mother to the station had been unable to find a parking space and just dropped her off, not understanding how confusing this would be for Mother.)

This stranger saw my mother's distress. She took the time and trouble to help her, to find out who needed to know, and to make the call to me.

LIZZIE, *daughter*

You think of some of your experiences and think, "How did I get through that?" You made it, and you think, "I'm okay." So it does give you some sense of accomplishment—you got through it.

MARILYN, *daughter*

As my mother became less able to take care of herself, I moved her from her hometown, Dallas, to mine in Colorado. It was necessary, but I felt terribly guilty, so I wanted to do something to make her very happy. I decided to have a family reunion in her honor. There was a total of twenty-eight people.

We had been close, but had drifted apart. Phone calls were rare. The planning gave everyone a new sense of purpose and a reason to call or e-mail. We were doing this for Mom. We were doing this because we were family.

The big weekend finally arrived. The next four days were re-markable. They changed my life. They taught me that there is nothing stronger and more precious and uplifting than the love and support of family.

The reunion was two years ago, but the phone calls and e-mails continue. This is my gift and my greatest joy. The ugliness of Alzheimer's brought us together again, with joy . . . with strength . . . with love.

LAURIE FRASIER, *daughter*

The gift Alzheimer's gives me is the gift of witnessing love in its el-emental form. Every day I witness such incredible love in mar-riages, families, and friendships. I try not to overlook that love. I think it's not just a gift to me, but it's the gift Alzheimer's gives to all of us, if only we stop to see it.

PAUL RAIA, *grandson, director of Patient and*
Family Support, Massachusetts Chapter of
the Alzheimer's Association

❧

If I had to single out only one gift, it would have to be the gift of faith. I was given the teaching and the strength and love that I needed to see us through this illness. When I ask for help and strength again, they will be given.

I can understand these gifts only as a grace, gifts from the source I call God. Caregiving taught me too much about my own limitations to take the credit myself. God is still a mystery way beyond my understanding, and my theology is a muddle, but nonetheless there are some deep truths I know now that have changed my life, even if I cannot put them into words.

As Words Fail

My dog understands every word I say. There would be a hole in our lives if she wasn't here.

Patient

Oh, I can't think of her name, but she's my favorite girl, almost.
KITTY, *patient, referring to a beloved daughter-in-law*

I could enjoy sharing with a small child his friendly nonverbal world in a way I could never have done before. Not only was my aphasia [difficulty finding words] not a problem—it was like the absence of street noise so I could better savor the music.

MORRIS FRIEDELL, *patient*

One of my oldest friends has Alzheimer's too. It is difficult for Pete to talk coherently, but last week we went to a concert together. Though he could not tell us what he was feeling, he gave every evidence of enjoying himself. This man, in his own way, is in touch with his environment, and his ingrained habits of courtesy carry him through.

JIM ANTHONY, *patient*

I know from the small glimpses of it that my mind has shown me so far that when I can no longer communicate with the world outside of my own mind, my brain will take me to a very peaceful calm gentle place.

It's a very peaceful, relaxing place where your mind just kind of drifts off and you become very unaware of your surroundings. Someday I know I'll be there all the time, but for now I still have a lot of work to do while I am still functional enough to fight going to that place. But as this disease progresses for me, I understand more and more what the caretakers are talking about as they describe their uncommunicative loved ones. I know they have just gone to this peaceful, relaxing place in their mind where you aren't bothered by what is happening around you. It's a place that I find myself starting to drift to more often myself.

DOREEN, *patient*

As Words Fail

. . .

Guessing what Rita is trying to say is a challenge. It's like playing charades.

RICHARD, *husband*

One evening my brother John taped the conversation when he and Dad were looking at an old photo album, pictures of his growing up and college years. I didn't play it until years later, when Dad could no longer talk—and suddenly, Dad was there again.

NANCY PETERSON, *daughter*

It hurts because you're wondering what's actually going on inside there—she really wants to try and just can't, and that's what hurts, the not knowing.

BELINDA, *daughter*

Vid often misnames things. He might say, "I can't find my stove," instead of "coat." When I respond, "You want to wear your stove?" Vid laughs, then I laugh, and we both feel better.

JANE, *wife*

175

There's nothing to do. We tried taking her out places, but that was hard on her because it confuses her. Just about all you can do is hug her and pat her and tell her you love her. And she'll take your face in her hands and say, "I love you too," but she has no idea who she is talking to. But I think she feels a sense of safety.

JOANNA, daughter

I would walk with my mother, and people would come up and say, "Well, is this your daughter?" And she would say, "Oh, this is my sister." And I'd say, "No, Mom, I'm your daughter." And she would look at me and say, "That's even better!"

MARILYN, daughter

I feel blessed that I can still do things for my wife. Yesterday, we went out to Quincy Market and shopped and had lunch. Those simple things now make a great day.

MIKE, husband

Sometimes I get impatient and feel very confined. Then it breaks through how hard it is for him, and I know my losses are less. It reminds me that we're on this journey together.

ANN DAVIDSON, wife

Hughes and I now share a new kind of intimacy, a nurturing unspoken kind that reaches out from the heart. My love for Hughes is stronger today than ever before. For the first time in our marriage, I understand the meaning of unconditional love.

LELA SHANKS, *wife*

My wife, Elizabeth, has been in the grip of Alzheimer's for nearly ten years. . . . It has been frustrating to me to hear her talk but not be able to decipher what she is saying because the words don't come out right. But one recent day, at lunchtime, she suddenly said, loud and clear, "I love you" . . . that made my day for a week! And the same "miracle" occurred the following week, when she uttered the same three little words.

JONATHAN SCHULKIN, *husband*

My brother-in-law had not spoken coherently for many months. But one day, when his small granddaughter started to climb up on the exercise machine, he suddenly called out, "Watch out!"

PHYLLIS, *sister-in-law*

I've said good-bye to my husband. I live with a two-year-old now.

ANN, *wife*

My father and I were very much alike—on the go, organizing things—and that father disappeared a long time ago. But I was able to get close to him in a new way. We'd take walks, I'd get a hug from him, some recognition, and it would mean so much.

NANCY PETERSON, *daughter*

I do believe this illness cannot destroy one's essence but only strikes at the surface, removing memories that form part of our exterior persona. Who we really are is not so easily destroyed.

GINETTE, *dementia researcher*

My relationship with my mother is more intimate than it ever was before. When I walk in to see her, her eyes light up. I've learned how to be with her, and this is a pure gift.

SUSAN BABCOCK, *daughter*

Once, when I went to visit my uncle, I was in the middle of a very painful breakup with my boyfriend. I talked and cried, telling him all about it. Pete couldn't talk, but he held my hand, and his eyes told me he cared.

KATHY, *great-niece*

I hadn't seen my mother for six months, since I live so far away, but I felt she recognized me as someone special to her. That's enough.

KIT, *daughter*

The last year and a half of my father's life were among the happiest. He wasn't lonely anymore, and even in his impaired state, he had tremendous joie de vivre. He would laugh with us about anything, even if he didn't understand the joke.

RUTH MACNAUGHTON, *daughter*

Though Mom was mostly mute during this stage and responded very little to life around her, she could still walk as long as I walked with her. She took to pacing almost constantly during the day, which meant I spent a good portion of the day pacing as well. . . . [None of the medications] seemed to help relax her.

One night, after many weeks of this behavior, I was growing more and more exasperated and exhausted . . . I snapped at her, "Mom . . . please sit down for at least five minutes or I'll go crazy." She looked at me more clearly than she had in several months and in an angry tone asked, "Would you like to trade places with me?"

I was stunned. All I could say was, "No, Mom. I'm sorry." "WELL THEN SIT DOWN AND SHUT UP!"

JEANNE PARSONS, *daughter*

❧

It was hard for us to make the shift from words to nonverbal communication. My husband and I had both been in love with words and cared about using them precisely. He taught English literature and composition for all of his working life;

I had been an English teacher and then a lawyer for a publishing company. But Pete gradually lost vocabulary, and it often was hard to guess how much he understood from our words. I began to learn that my tone of voice and manner were often more important than my words, and to act calm when I was in turmoil. I didn't always succeed, but the disease did wonders for my skills as an actress.

I missed Pete's words the most when something was wrong, and he couldn't tell us what it was and we couldn't guess. But it was wonderful when we connected without words.

Placement

In the beginning, I didn't know what people meant by "placement." It's when a family "places" the patient in a nursing home or assisted living. I grew to hate the term—and not just because I knew it would be difficult and painful if we had to take that step. It sounded so impersonal, like deciding where to place a piece of furniture, and yet it was too personal—it was clear that I would be doing the placing. This would not be a joint decision. In fact, I shrank from the term not only through the placement process but afterward—I would talk of my husband's "move," and I still do. Taking that step was the hardest thing I have ever done.

It was hard to see friends from the support group deteriorate and go into placement. It was hard for me to watch this happen to them because I know that someday it will probably happen to me.

JOHN DURAND, *patient*

One of the things that I've come to understand is that not everyone realizes that there is no reason for me to delay going into a nursing home any longer than necessary. The only thing necessary is for me to find a home now for my cat.

After that I can go into a nursing home as soon as it is time. And that isn't a bad thing. Given how difficult it is becoming for me to live alone, I welcome being in a place where someone can take the responsibilities of daily life (food, clothes, etc.) off of me. Where I don't have to try to figure out what to eat, what to wear, to clean clothes, etc.

DOREEN, *patient*

❧

I knew I should start visiting local Alzheimer's units, but I just couldn't face it. I was blown away when my friend Sally—someone with no close experience with Alzheimer's or nursing homes—offered to go with me.

In the end, I went instead with another member of the support group, but it was Sally's offer that got me "unstuck."

Betsy, just *do it*. Dad would hate to be putting you through this
kind of pain.

NANCY, *daughter*

You know, it would have been appropriate to place your husband
when I first met him—and that was three years ago.

DR. LEWIS LEVY, *primary physician*

So is the question whether you place him now—or six months
from now?

A wise listener

Why do these places choose fruity names that just make it harder?
"Renaissance"! "Golden Age"! "Sunrise"! I'm going to open a unit
called "Sunset."

DOROTHY, *wife*

Is it a contest how long you keep him at home?

JOIE, *wife*

My doctor told me I had two choices—to find full-time help or arrange my funeral.

TED DISTLER, *husband*

Minnie Mae, as we all do, feared the nursing home, but she didn't resist her new home. She seems to know that she needs more care than Dot Benson and I could provide.

I was less accepting. I resisted our separation until the day her new life began. On the first day, I stood at a distance for the first time and saw how much patience and skill she needs. In the middle of her caretaking, Dot and I denied the seriousness of the changes and the way they were accelerating.

DONALD MURRAY, *husband*

Mom told me she got lost in the neighborhood she has lived in for the last forty years. And it was just crossing the alley. Am I a schmuck to put her in a retirement community?

SAM, *son*

"Placement"? It feels like murder.

MARTY, *wife*

186

I had to learn the difference between custodial care and relational care. Others can provide custodial care, but I was the only one who could maintain the relationship. When I recognized that managing the custodial care had become damaging to my relationship with Jim, I could accept that it was time to change the care plan. It would have been tragic to lose that relationship while it could still grow.

PAM, *wife*

❧

For the first few days I felt mostly relief and thankfulness that we had found such a loving place for my husband. I was exhausted and began to catch up on sleep; I reveled in the freedom from the daily pressures and uncertainties. Then I suddenly realized how much I was hating it—at the same time. I missed seeing Pete every day. I missed snuggling up to him in bed. I missed the comforts of getting his dinner, helping him get dressed, seeing that he brushed his teeth. By then, most of our interaction had been around these simple physical acts. It was hard to rely so completely on strangers—especially when they could not tend to him as promptly as I had been able to at home.

Life Goes On

You know, one thing I haven't figured out about this place . . . no one ever seems to *graduate* from here.

JAMES NICHOLS, *patient, a scholar and professor*

Once I'm dead, the only thing that will matter is, did I continue to work at leaving the world a better place than I found it. And I can do that as easily in a nursing home as I can here at home . . . there is no question at all in my mind that for as long as I am able to communicate in any way at all, I can be helpful to others in a nursing home.

And that's all that matters, not where I physically am but am I doing the one and only thing that matters for any of us . . . doing my best to leave the world a better place than I found it.

DOREEN, *patient*

◆   ◆   ◆

Are we going to visit the Nervous Home today?

Young great-granddaughter

Some people see my daily visits to Felicity as a burden or sacrifice. Instead, my seeing her so often is a venting of my pent-up gratitude; I feel distressed when I can't see her. Impaired as she is, she still gives us parts of her old self. She's funny and she's responsive to our humor. When she bursts into song on my arrival on the ward, what greater reward can I have, short of her miraculous recovery?

DANIEL, *husband*

I now realize I tried to keep my husband at home too long. The change to a nursing home was a great relief for *him,* not just for me. He was now in a setting he could manage. No one asked him to try to do things he couldn't do. He was no longer surrounded by reminders of a lost past. There was always help at hand.

And for me, it was almost like a second honeymoon. Managing the home health aides and all the rest necessary for his physical care was an enormous stress. Once I passed that burden to the nursing home, we could both enjoy just being together.

PAM KUNKEMUELLER, *wife*

Life Goes On

Margaret is quite unaware of her surroundings and seems quite content, which is a great relief. I was so fearful that, when the day did come that she would need constant surveillance and nursing care, she would miss me and home and the dogs—thankfully she doesn't.

ADRIAN, *husband*

She'd sit there and talk (make gibberish sounds) and it was beautiful to see the other residents say, "Oh, really?" We were carrying on this make-believe situation that she really felt a part of.

BELINDA, *daughter*

Our marriage was so close—no secrets—that the chapters run together. We read the chronicle of one life, not two.

But our new chapter is, for the first time, not a collaboration. We live a few miles apart—I in a condo, she in a nursing home where the doors are always locked . . . We listen to each other, but we cannot often understand the accounts of the foreign lives we now inhabit . . .

But our lives are not quite separate. We may not speak but simply hold hands. We simply hang on against the inevitable future. For the moment, holding hands, we become one person after all.

DONALD MURRAY, *husband*

❧

When people asked, "Does he still know you?" I wanted to hit them. Don't they have any idea how painful that is?

I would struggle to reply calmly, usually saying, "His daughter and I believe he still recognizes us as someone very special to him." To closer friends I might add that the recognition was a bit slow to come. We had both learned that he would draw back if we tried to hug him as soon as we arrived, but often welcome a hug a few minutes later.

That question doesn't bother me. It shows that the person asking the question understands the magnitude of what we're dealing with.

MARSHA, *daughter*

It's the only question most people can think of. I take it in stride.

DOROTHY, *wife*

It is VERY hard to visit Ed. I think his anxiety increases when I am there because he immediately starts worrying about when I am going to leave. My daughters are giving me a hard time; they don't think I am spending enough time there. I am emotionally drained every time I leave the place, and I don't think my kids understand that.

JUDY, *wife*

This was a lesson I had to learn over and over with my father's illness, even up to the end: that it would be progressive no matter what I did, that he would get worse no matter what I did. I think this is the hardest lesson about Alzheimer's disease for a caregiver: you can never do enough to make a difference in the course of the disease. Hard because what we feel anyway is that we have never *done* enough. We blame ourselves. . . . In the end, all those judgments, those self-judgments, are pointless. The disease is inexorable, cruel. It scoffs at everything.

SUE MILLER, *daughter*

Some people tell my father he should not visit my mother in the nursing home so often and that he should take up other activities. He does do other things, but visiting my mother almost every day is what he needs to do.

KIT, *daughter*

My mother has lost so much understanding of her past—so many crucial defining events and relationships are gone—but with the lack of awareness has come greater serenity and happiness for her. She is enjoying her life now and is no longer in the grip of fear and anxiety, and for this we are very grateful.

JUDITH, *daughter*

It's such a big mystery, living in suspended animation like this. But there is a kind of grace involved. . . . When you do something for someone with Alzheimer's, they forget it as soon as it's done, so you know you're not doing it for credit. It's a kind of sacrament. You do it because of all the things that have been done for you, maybe not even by the parent you are caring for.

COURTENAY, *daughter*

It was a long drive to see my mother-in-law, five or six hours, so we couldn't go very often. We would do things like looking at photographs with her to call forth what she used to know. She would try to dredge up memories to please us, but we wondered if we were forcing her to go deep into a part of herself that she had "lost" or was trying to protect, a part she would have to put away again when we left. Was this for our benefit or hers? Clearly we were the ones pleading for response. We never knew what our visits cost her, or whether she felt abandoned when we left, or whether it was even fair to call forth such effort when we could not be with her more.

FAITH, *daughter-in-law*

We lament for people who tell us how "terrible" it is that he "isn't himself" anymore. He still gives me a lot. I guess the things that they think are missing in him are all the things that made him who he was. Past tense. He didn't stop giving and we haven't stopped taking what he gives.

ERIC HUGHES SHANKS, *son*

He wakes up happy every morning. What more could I ask?

DEBBIE, *wife, and an Episcopal priest*

Everything here is stable, except perhaps my emotions. I struggle to keep a positive outlook and to stop dwelling on the negatives. Such a struggle!

JOIE, *wife*

I will never forget watching Pete enjoy an ice cream cone today. Such attention, and such enormous satisfaction! It was a privilege to witness.

Augusta, *friend*

❦

Pete lived at Sunrise for more than two years, so Nancy Lee and I had time to become fond of other residents and the staff. Some visits felt like the Mad Hatter's tea party; others brought a blessed interval of peace. I would arrive with nerves jangling after a hectic day and rush-hour traffic but would leave calmly, restored by such simple things as tossing a ball with Pete, getting a hug from Bernie, or looking at a picture book with Ollie. And by seeing love in action as the staff cared for the residents with patience and compassion. They seemed never to lose their sense of humor or their respect for each resident.

During the last few months, however, it became harder for me to connect with Pete. It was hard, too, to persuade myself that the problem was the disease, not me. It felt too much like my own failure. I kept thinking of a friend in the support group who felt she connected with her husband's soul more deeply than ever before. Was she just lucky, or was I doing something wrong? Was it that she could see her husband almost every day and I could not? Or was it just that the damage to her husband's brain was different from the damage to Pete's? Eventually, most of the time, I stopped trying to match her experience and began to accept our own reality. Pete might not show a response, but I loved him deeply and knew he loved me. I was doing my best. And the disease would have its own way, no matter how hard we tried.

As the End Approaches

Stan is in an easier place now. He's not unhappy anymore, he's not happy, either—he just is. It's easier for him, and therefore for me.

JOIE, *wife*

On a day when she's not hardly responding, I feel she's gone, the mother I know. I almost wish it's over. Then all it takes is one good day, where she smiles and says this, and you want to hang on. And that's when you really feel the loss.

JENNY, *daughter*

It's a roller-coaster, a real roller-coaster.

MARILYN, *daughter*

It helps me to remember that Dad is eighty-five—with or without Alzheimer's.

TOM, *son*

The worst was that she was a singer, and we would sing at the nursing home, and when she could no longer sing in key, she died a week or two later. I probably grieved more that day she wasn't singing on key than I grieved when she died, because that was the last part of her still together.

MARGIE, *daughter*

The last few months of my mother's life were in some ways the best in our relationship. She had been very demanding all of her life, but now she was open in a way she had never been before. We became closer than I imagined we could.

MARSHA, *daughter*

We are like many other families who come to the bedside of a loved one and look into eyes that no longer flicker with recognition. It rearranges your universe. It strips away everything but the most important truth: that the soul is alive, even if the mind is faltering.

PATTI DAVIS, *daughter of Ronald Reagan*

I think we're agreed that if she gets pneumonia, we won't treat it— but the decision to treat or not to treat is the hardest.

ISABELLE MCNAIR, *daughter*

I had gone to spend an evening with Pete every week or two while he was still at home and went to see him in the residential unit as often as I could. But I couldn't bear to go see him at the very end, when he was dying. I needed to keep my earlier happier memories.

KATHY, *great-niece*

As the Alzheimer's progressed, I clung desperately to each stage of the disease: the sleeping and forgetting one; the wandering one; the sleepless and the distracted one. Each stage became a sort of friend. But now, this last stage—feeding Iris with a spoon, kissing her when she consents to take a drink—seems to have abandoned us.

JOHN BAYLEY, *husband*

The point is that as awful as Alzheimer's is, *it is just another way to die.* . . . There is no hierarchy of what is a worst death. What matters isn't how we die . . . what matters is how we are treated, regarded, considered, and cared for during the process.

BEVERLY BIGTREE MURPHY, *wife*

201

A wise counselor once asked a group of Alzheimer's wives if we felt like widows. It was, at the time, a startling question, but I recognized the similarities: I was already in charge of the household, and I was trying to ease the losses in Pete's companionship by building new friendships and keeping busy. So I had, for some years, thought of myself as a something-percent widow. Perhaps a 50 percent widow at the time of that conversation; a jump to 80 percent when Pete moved to assisted living and I lived alone again; gradually increasing to the 90s in the last few months. But the day before he died I began to understand that being a 100 percent widow would be very different.

Final Days

The last time the hospice aide tried to feed Hughes, he stated plainly, "Leave me alone."

I had never seen anyone die before, and I had no idea what to expect. But Hughes "told me." In the last two or three weeks of his life, he withdrew from me and into himself in a way that told me he was moving on to another world.

Two days before his death, I wanted desperately to get some recognition from him—anything. . . . On an impulse, I asked him, "Honey, will you be my guardian angel?" And to my great surprise, he bowed his head in the affirmative . . . and did so again twice later.

LELA SHANKS, *wife*

I wasn't gone thirty minutes, and I was really upset that he didn't wait for me. After all those years, I missed out, and to this day I feel cheated. But I also understand that perhaps he needed to do it without me. That perhaps it was easier for him to go without me there.

BEVERLY BIGTREE MURPHY, *wife*

Iris died on February 8, 1999. She had grown steadily weaker. Without bother or fuss, as if someone she trusted had helped her come to a decision, she stopped eating and drinking. During the last week, she took to opening her blue eyes very wide, as if merrily.

JOHN BAYLEY, *husband*

The doctor doubted that Betty's husband would last long enough for either the son or the daughter, overseas in the military, to arrive. A day later, after the son arrived, he told the family that he couldn't understand it. Her husband wasn't getting worse but he also wasn't improving. Two days later the daughter arrived at the hospital. She walked into the room, kissed her father, told him she loved him. The rest of the family gathered in the room and shortly after, he died.

BEVERLY BIGTREE MURPHY, *wife*

I wanted my husband to die at home—and he did, but his home then was the nursing home where the staff had loved him and cared for both of us for many months.

PAM KUNKEMUELLER, *wife*

All the grief I'd held in for days—really, for years—poured out of me. I didn't care how loud I was.

SUE MILLER, *daughter*

My reaction and my curiosity were a surprise to me, a pleasant surprise. Dead was different. Dead was quiet. Dead was peaceful and dead was curious, but dead was not scary.

SALLY CALLAHAN, *daughter*

It's more of a change than I expected. All I can feel right now is glad that he doesn't have to do this anymore.

DOROTHY, *wife*

I see now that when you're dead, you're really dead.

IRENE FRANZEN, *wife*

❧

After so many years of gradual decline, I almost stopped wondering when it would end. Even when Pete went into hospice care, the nurse doing the evaluation thought it might be an "early admit"—in other words, he might survive beyond the six-month guideline for hospice eligibility. Instead, he took us all by surprise and died three weeks later. I felt almost as much bewilderment as sorrow. We had known for so long this day would come: how could it still be such a shock and seem to come so fast?

Pete had never been slow to take action, and clearly he had physical discomfort during those last weeks. By then the damage to his brain and body was severe, but I couldn't help believing that he had nonetheless made his final decision: enough!

Afterward

We can be sad now, but not so anxious about what was to come.

KIT, *daughter*

At the funeral, one of my relatives came up and said, "At last!" I know she meant to express sympathy for our years of strain and sorrow, and yes, we did feel relief. But somehow it was absolutely the wrong thing to say.

EVE, *wife*

People expect me to be crying all the time, but I'm not. Yes, I miss Stan badly, but I'm glad the hard part is over for him. There were lots of tears in the beginning, but we could talk about it, and we took the bull by the horns. Alzheimer's gave us time for closure. And I am thankful we had such a good marriage.

JOIE, *wife*

If asked, I would do this all over, knowing what I know now. I have to say I wouldn't have missed Tom Murphy for all the world. He's given me more than anyone could imagine.

BEVERLY BIGTREE MURPHY, *wife*

Grief and relief—you have to hold onto and honor both parts of what you are experiencing now.

JEANNE SMITH, MD

Mom died on May 6. I have not been able to cry until now. Now, two months later, the tears won't stop.

Daughter

I don't think I cried for three months. I cried at the moment he died but not at the wake. I was completely numb; all I could feel was relief and thank God every day that it was over.

IRENE, *daughter*

After Milly passed, I found that coming out of it was not as easy as I thought. I found myself withdrawing even more, and it took great effort to get out into the "other" world.

BUBBLEHEAD

Afterward

I'd had a difficult relationship with my mother. Her dying seemed endless and her existence pointless, and at times I felt as if once again she'd never do what we wanted her to do. I kept asking myself, "Why doesn't she die?" But after she died I could see that this long dying was a time of healing for both of us. I could hold her hand and sing to her and read psalms, and I think she felt loved as well. This time with her was a gift, for all of its difficulty, and I'm a different person because of it.

CARL, *son*

There is a sense of what I call empty hands. What can I do now? I've been a caregiver for many years—now I have no care to give!

SUE, *daughter*

Why do I stay with the Alzheimer List chat room? I need to know what the hell happened! I was too busy LIVING with Mother's Alzheimer's, coping and adjusting, finding what worked, unraveling the layers within layers of this obscene disease to have time to allow my grief-anger-RAGE emotions to surface. The seventeen months Mother was here with me were a whirlwind with no time to stop and LOOK.

HCASTON, *daughter*

These days I'm thinking a lot about what I could have, SHOULD have done along the way. As I look back in my grief, for every one thing I might have done right, I feel like I did 1,000 things wrong. How could she have placed such trust in me?

Daughter

For many of us, the grief is that our loved ones have had to suffer so long with dementia, while we get to watch. For us, death is a blessing for the loved one and a comfort for those left behind. Missing them after they are gone seems a small price to pay to NOT see them suffer every day.

Daughter

For me, I think the grief was much worse during the illness than it has been since he's been gone. And even though he's only been dead a year and a half, I have to go back eight years to think that I had a father.

IRENE, *daughter*

Afterward

The thing is that the grieving before they die wears you out. You're just worn out. So when they finally die, you're just relieved that you don't have to do that all day anymore.

JUNE, *daughter*

For two years following the death of my mother, I viewed the care-giving period of my life through half-closed eyes. I guess I was trying to shield my soul and my conscience. It is painful to go back and look at one's stupid and thoughtless mistakes, but I knew I had no other choice. I had to hold this ball of grief in my hand and examine it before I could go on with my life.

SUE, *daughter*

This year I'm acutely aware of how lonely I am for her. It's almost as if last year didn't count; the grief was such a constant companion that I couldn't be "lonely." In an odd way, it was a comfort to be grief-filled. This year there isn't that protection. Time to be a Grown Up, I suppose.

Daughter

I now live my life as if I expect to get Alzheimer's by the time I am sixty-five. I stopped working, began teaching yoga and providing Reiki (energy healing) in the hopes that by being in good health, I will avoid getting the disease. I have spent time with my husband who is retired now and with both our mothers who have their medical issues. I try to live life fully and to enjoy what I do each moment. I think I am more balanced.

LEIGH, *daughter*

If there is one thing this experience has taught me, it's to live life today and do not even look ahead. I try to live every day full today and have no fears for tomorrow, because it's not guaranteed to any of us.

IRENE, *daughter*

❧

I would never have believed this could be true, but sometimes I miss the intensity of the caregiving years. It was a time of living close to the core of life.

Sources

PROFILES

Here's a little more background on some of the voices in this book.

Bernie Shapiro thought it was "just old age" when he first noticed problems remembering and pronouncing words, although he was only sixty-seven. As the situation got worse over time, he sought a diagnosis. It was a devastating shock to get the verdict of probable Alzheimer's. He credits his wife Barbara and the Massachusetts Chapter of the Alzheimer's Association for pulling him out of despair and into "life beyond the diagnosis."

Dave Harris, a former airline pilot, lives in Boise, Idaho. He too went into a serious depression as he struggled to accept the diagnosis, but then sought counseling and antidepressants. He got invaluable help from other patients and the Alzheimer's Association. He now serves as a director of the Idaho chapter of the Association and of an interdenominational program called Faith in Action, which recruits, trains, and coordinates volunteers to provide respite care for Alzheimer's patients and frail elders.

Bill Orme-Johnson had to retire at fifty-eight because of memory problems. Bill was a biochemist, a researcher and faculty member at the Massachusetts Institute of Technology. At the time of diagnosis, Bill and Carol had four children still at home (the eldest was eleven). Seven years later, still playing his guitar, Bill moved to a specialized Alzheimer's assisted living facility, partly because of another illness.

Dorothy and Norman Dahl enjoyed years of happy and busy retirement before Norman began to lose his zest and forget things. His diagnosis for the first few years was depression, not dementia. I didn't meet Norman until he was an eighty-year-old with Alzheimer's but, oh! that smile. I fell in love with him on the spot.

Pam Kunkemueller describes her marriage to Jim as a "fifties classic": Dad at work, Mom at home. He made the money, she spent it. Then Jim's business started running into trouble. Jim was only in his fifties, so it took years to recognize that he was suffering from a rare dementia, eventually identified as Progressive Supranuclear Palsy. Pam now volunteers for the Alzheimer's Association, co-leading a support group and serving on the Chapter's help line and board.

Marsha Mirkin met a double challenge: both parents, Sidney and Ann, suffered from Alzheimer's. She also faced the demands of caregiving from afar, as she lives near Boston and her parents were in Florida until the last year of their lives. Marsha is a clinical psychologist, a resident scholar at the Brandeis University Women's Studies Research Center, and author of *The Women Who Dance by the Sea: Finding Ourselves in the Stories of Our Biblical Foremothers.*

"Kit" also suffered the difficulties of distance. Her parents were in Arizona; she works for a publisher on the east coast. Kit, however, took comfort in her father's care of her mother.

Carl and Faith Scovel thought they could care for Carl's mother at home. After one week, during which she kept escaping and wandering into unfamiliar city streets, the family had to move her to a nursing home instead. Carl is Minister Emeritus of King's Chapel in Boston.

Jim Anthony was a close friend of ours long before any of us worried about Alzheimer's. For most of his career he was an English teacher and a gifted (but unpublished) poet. As my husband's illness progressed, Jim would sometimes come to spend the evening with Pete and give me a break. A few years later Jim started having problems himself, but it was several years before he got the diagnosis of Alzheimer's at age fifty-nine. He lives with his partner, Bruce Steiner.

The Noonan family carries a rare genetic mutation predisposing them to Alzheimer's. They are one of a few hundred families world-wide to suffer such a high risk. The disease has directly attacked three of the ten siblings and afflicts the others with repeated loss and high risk. Four of them speak in this book: patients Fran Noonan Powers and Butch Noonan and their siblings Eryc Noonan and Julie Lawson Noonan. The family fights back by organizing a Memory Ride that has raised hundreds of thousands of dollars for research. They also volunteer as research subjects and educate others. The family was featured in *The Forgetting*, a PBS special on Alzheimer's.

Chip Gerber was a social worker and an advocate for the elderly, and now his advocacy for Alzheimer's includes testifying before Congress. He and his wife, Sharon, formerly of Ohio, now live in Florida. His sense of humor pervades his online journal, "My Journey," which can be found at www.zarcrom.com/users/alzheimers/chip.

JanMina is the Internet name chosen by Jan Phillips, a Californian. She and her mother have both been diagnosed with Alzheimer's, which shapes Jan's advocacy for a cure. Her writings are quoted on various Internet sites, and her home page is www.ycsi.net/users/laura/janmina.html.

Morris Friedell was diagnosed with Alzheimer's soon after retiring as a sociology professor at the University of California, Santa Barbara. He co-founded DASNI, where he met his new wife, Andrea. They live in Houston, Texas. His Web site at www.members.aol.com/MorrisFF includes provocative essays as well as an autobiography.

Alice Young, mother of five, writes of beautiful summers on a Minnesota lake and of the difficulties of moving from her home in Florida to an assisted living center near her daughters in Indiana. Her home page is at www.geocities.com/allieyoung1.

Doreen gives extraordinary reports of her experience with a dementia diagnosed as Pick's Disease. Because she lived alone (with her cats), she chose to enter a nursing home while she still retained many skills.

There she has been able to continue her passion for animals, spending many hours caring for the home's pets and aviary. Her site includes journal entries and illuminating comments on "Life Changes." www.homestead.com/ftdpicksdisease.

FOR FURTHER READING

From Patients

Chip, JanMina, Morris, Alice, and Doreen give detailed reports on their Web sites. They are all members of DASNI, an online advocacy and support group for people with a diagnosis of dementia. The DASNI site, www.dasninternational.org, offers links to Web sites of other patients too.

Thomas DeBaggio. Reprinted with the permission of The Free Press, a Division of Simon & Schuster Adult Publishing Group. From *Losing My Mind: An Intimate Look at Life with Alzheimer's.* Copyright © 2002 by Thomas DeBaggio. All rights reserved.

Jeanne Lee. *Just Love Me, My Life Turned Upside Down by Alzheimer's,* West Lafayette, IN: Purdue University Press, 2003.

See also *Speaking Our Minds: Personal Reflections from Individuals with Alzheimer's,* by Lisa Snyder. New York: W.H. Freeman and Company, 1999. Lengthy interviews with seven patients, including Bea, Betty, Bill, Bob, and Jean.

From Family Members

The quotations from these family members come from their books or articles.

Terry Baltz, from *Fierce Blessing: A Journey Into Alzheimer's, Compassion, and the Joy of Being*, by Wayne and Terry Baltz. Red Feather Lakes, CO: Prairie Divide Press, 2003.

John Bayley, "Last Jokes," *The New Yorker*, August 2, 1999.

Sally Callahan, *My Mother's Voice*. Forest Knolls, CA: Elder Books, 2000.

Eleanor Cooney, *Death in Slow Motion*. New York: HarperCollins, 2003.

Joanne Koenig Coste, also quoting Bernie Reisman, Bill, and Jason. From *Learning to Speak Alzheimer's* by Joanne Koenig Coste. Copyright © 2003 by Joanne Koenig Coste. Reprinted by permission of Houghton Mifflin Company. All rights reserved.

Ann Davidson, *San Francisco Chronicle,* September 30, 2001; *Alzheimer's, a Love Story: One Year in My Husband's Journey*, Birch Lane Press, 1997.

Jonathan Franzen, also quoting his mother Irene Franzen, "My Father's Brain," in *How to Be Alone: Essays*, New York: Picador, 2003.

Robertson McQuilkin, *A Promise Kept: The Story of an Unforgettable Love*. Carol Stream, IL: Tyndale House Publishers, 1998.

Sources

Sue Miller, also quoting James Nichols. From *The Story of My Father: A Memoir* by Sue Miller, copyright © 2003 by Sue Miller. Used by permission of Alfred A. Knopf, a division of Random House, Inc.

Beverly Bigtree Murphy, from her Web site, bigtreemurphy.com and *He Used to Be Somebody: A Journey into Alzheimer's Disease Through the Eyes of a Caregiver*, Boulder CO: Gibbs Associates, 1995.

Donald Murray, "When One Life Becomes Two," *Boston Globe,* June 15, 2004.

Charles Pierce, excerpted by permission from *Hard to Forget: An Alzheimer's Story.* Copyright © 2000 by Charles P. Pierce.

Lela Knox Shanks, also quoting Cedric Shanks, Christopher Shanks, and Shela Omell Richards. Reprinted from *Your Name Is Hughes Hannibal Shanks: A Caregiver's Guide to Alzheimer's,* by Lela Knox Shanks by permission of the University of Nebraska Press, © 1996 by the University of Nebraska Press.

Daphne Simpkins, "No Regrets," Christian Century, November 1, 2003, adapted from *The Long Goodnight: My Father's Journey into Alzheimer's.* Grand Rapids, MI: William B. Eerdmans, 2003.

From *Finding the Joy in Alzheimer's: Caregivers Share the Joyful Times,* 2002, by Brenda Avadian, MA, Editor, North Star Books. Excerpted and abridged by permission from Brenda Avadian and Laurie Frasier, "Four Special Days"; Jeanne Parsons, from "Sit Down and Shut Up" and "She's Much Nicer Than You Are"; and Jonathan Schulkin, from "Those Three Words."

From Other Sources

"I'm Still Here," a handout of patient comments collected by Elaine Silverio of the Massachusetts Chapter of the Alzheimer's Association.

"Brilliant Insights," a handout of patient comments collected by Sally Ollerton of the Cleveland Chapter of the Alzheimer's Association.

From newsletters of the Massachusetts Chapter of the Alzheimer's Association (some available online at www.alzmass.org): James Anthony, "Ask Dr. Know: A Special Guest Column by Someone Who's Been There" Summer/Fall 1997, Volume 15, Number 3; Cathleen McBride, "Setting a New Stage," Summer 2003, Volume 21, Number 3; Pamela Kunkemueller, "A Caregiver's Odyssey," Spring/Summer 1998, Volume 16, Numbers 1–2; Paul Raia quoted in "Upside to Caregiving," Fall 2003, Volume 21, Number 4.

Family Care Guide, May 1988 (first edition). The Massachusetts Chapter of the Alzheimer's Association published an updated edition in 2002, quoting C.K., S.G., M.S., and T.S.

The Caregiver Grief Study, a research project conducted by Dr. Thomas Meuser and Dr. Samuel Marwit. Tom and Sam kindly gave me some quotations from the focus groups, changing the names of the participants. (For more information on the study, see "Grief" in the Resources section.)

The Forgetting, PBS special, January 21, 2004. Comments from Edna Ballard, Harry Fuget, Lisa Gwyther, Butch Noonan, Isabelle Mc-Nair, and Frances Noonan Powers. See also David Shenk, *The Forgetting, Alzheimer's: Portrait of an Epidemic*. New York: Doubleday, 2001, quoting Ralph Waldo Emerson, C.S.H., and N.B.

"DASNI People in the News," www.dasninternational.org, stories quoting Marilyn, Ruth Harris, Lynn Jackson, Brian McNaughton, and Ben Stevens.

From online chat groups, notably "The Alzheimer List," an e-mail support group at alzheimer.wustl.edu/adrc2/alzheimerlist and the Anger Wall at www.alzwell.com. These include comments from Bubblehead, Dale, dayin, hcaston, Sam, and Zinnia.

"Memories Unmoored," by Priscilla Grant, *Smith Alumnae Quarterly*, Winter 2001–2002, quoting Howard Carew, Susan Babcock, Ruth MacNaughton, and Nancy Peterson.

Frank Carlino, "Morning Edition," National Public Radio November 13, 2002.

Patti Davis, "Our Family Today," *People*, December 15, 2003

Ted Distler quoted in *Advances*, the Alzheimer's Association Newsletter, Vol. 22 No. 4, Winter 2003.

Shelley Fabares, in "The Vanishing," *People*, February 27, 1995.

Lauri Covington Grantham, "Coffee, Cookies, and Goodbyes," www.alz.org/resources/shortstories, posted February 10, 2003.

Dave Harris, panel at Alzheimer's Public Policy Forum, March 2004.

Cary Henderson, quoted by Morris Friedell. www.members.aol.com/MorrisFF.

Harriet Hodgson, also quoting Don Bliss, *The Alzheimer's Caregiver: Dealing with the Realities of Dementia.* Minneapolis: Chronimed Publishing, 1998.

Julie Noonan Lawson quoted by Carol Wogrin. *Matters of Life and Death: Finding the Words to Say Goodbye.* New York: Broadway Books, 2001.

Mary Lockhart, "Mary's Page," www.ycsi.net/users/laura/mari5113.html.

Molly Ivins, also quoting Courtenay, "Caring About Chronic Care," *Boston Globe*, November 24, 1999.

Doug Manning, "Grief and Alzheimer's," www.insightbooks.com.

Edward J. Markey, Congressman from Massachusetts, speech to Alzheimer's Association, April 2, 2001.

Genny McGlynn quoted in *North Country Times* (nctimes.com/news/2001/20010513).

Bill Orme-Johnson, "A Surprising and Cruel Blow," *Boston Globe*, April 8, 2001.

Nina P. quoted in *Lessons Learned: Shared Experiences in Coping*, by participants of Duke University Support Groups, edited by Edna L. Ballard and Cornelia M. Poer.

Michael Reagan quoted in "A bold voice silenced" by Michael R. Blood and John Rogers, *Boston Globe*, June 13, 2004.

Ronald Reagan, letter to the American people, November 5, 1994.

Marty Saunders and Leigh Saunders Kitcher quoted by Richard Knox, "Growing Older," *Boston Globe*, November 10, 1997.

Sargent Shriver quoted in *Parade, The Sunday Newspaper Magazine*, October 26, 2003.

Margie Slyne quoted in "Centers of Support," *West Roxbury Transcript*, Massachusetts, November 18, 1998.

Gloria Sterin quoted in "Brilliant Insights."

And last, but especially dear to me, the friends, acquaintances and family who have shared their experiences. Jim Anthony, John Durand, Lewis Law, and Pam Kunkemueller gave me copies of their speeches for the Massachusetts Chapter of the Alzheimer's Association. Other contributions are from Henrietta Amadon, Jenneke Barton, Richard Conti, John and Peggi Durand, Dottie Evans, Stan Evans, Kit Everts, Betty Falsey, Joie Gerrish, Penelope Johnson, Wyn Kelley, Lewis and Margaret Law, Cathleen and Owen McBride, Lindsay McGinnis, Loretta Norris, Kathy O'Donnell, Mary and Terry O'Toole, Adrian

Pelly, John Peterson, Nancy Lee Peterson, Debbie Phillips, Carl and Faith Scovel, Margie Slyne, Judith Siporin, Claudia Stearns, Bruce Steiner, Bart Thomas, Jane Venckauskas, Lois Wasoff, Annette, Augusta, Chris, Colby, "Daniel," Ginette, Gisela, Jacob, Judy, "Kit," Nick, and the anonymous teenagers.

Selected Resources and Issues

ORGANIZATIONS

Four organizations offer extraordinarily comprehensive resources. They discuss many of the same issues, of course, but differ considerably in how they organize and present the information.

Alzheimer's Association
www.alz.org
800-272-3900; 312-335-8700
919 North Michigan Avenue, Suite 1100
Chicago, IL 60611-1676

The Alzheimer's Association has many local chapters, which offer educational programs, support groups, newsletters, and other resources. The 800 number provides a hotline staffed twenty-four hours a day. The Alzheimer's Association Web site provides links to local chapters, as well as an extraordinary variety of useful resources. The Web site is organized to help patients, families, or health professionals quickly find the materials most relevant to their perspective.

The Alzheimer's Association publishes more than one hundred fact sheets and short brochures addressing specific topics, many available online. Those of general interest include the following:

- Ten Warning Signs of Alzheimer's Disease
- Overview of Alzheimer's Disease and Related Dementias
- Living with Early-Onset Dementia
- You Can Make a Difference: 10 Ways to Help an Alzheimer Family
- Caregiver Stress: Signs to Watch For . . . Steps to Take
- How to Be a Long-Distance Caregiver
- Steps to Understanding Legal Issues
- Steps to Understanding Financial Issues

Other fact sheets and brochures discuss specific dementias, medications, research developments, behavioral issues, driving, taxes, and many other topics, ranging through all stages of the illness, from pre-diagnosis to choosing a nursing home and end-of-life issues like hospice.

Some brochures are available in Spanish, Chinese, and Korean. Check "Resources" for fact sheets, brochures, a Diversity Toolbox, and resource lists on specific topics. It is also possible to search the entire catalog of the Green-Field Library and Resource Center.

Alzheimer Society of Canada/Société Alzheimer du Canada
www.alzheimer.ca
800-616-8816 (only in Canada)
20 Eglinton Avenue, W., Suite 1200
Toronto, ON M4R 1KB

Like its U.S. counterpart, the Alzheimer Society of Canada offers local chapters and a rich variety of resources—in French as well as in English. The site includes a thoughtful discussion of ethical issues (see "Ethical Guidelines").

ADEAR—Alzheimer's Disease Education and Referral Center
www.alzheimers.org
800-438-4380
ADEAR Center

P.O. Box 8250
Silver Spring, MD 20907-8250

ADEAR is a service of the National Institute on Aging, one of the institutes within the U.S. Department of Health and Human Services. It strives to provide current, comprehensive, and unbiased information about Alzheimer's. It offers free publications, a caregiver's guide, referrals to support and research centers, information on clinical trials, searches of the literature, and will answer specific questions.

DASNI—Dementia Advocacy and Support Network International, www.dasninternational.org.

DASNI is a Web-based nonprofit organization of people diagnosed with dementia. Its purpose is "to promote respect and dignity for persons with dementia, provide a forum for the exchange of information, encourage support mechanisms such as local groups, counseling, and Internet linkages, and to advocate for services."

DASNI offers a chatroom for persons with dementia, and the site includes links to Web sites of people with dementia and to other resources.

INITIAL STEPS AFTER DIAGNOSIS

- *First Steps for Families* from the Alzheimer Society of Canada, www.alzheimer.ca.
- *What Shall I Do if It Is AD?* www.agelessdesign.com/FAQ includes suggestions from patient JanMina.

FOR PEOPLE WITH DEMENTIA

The national sites offer some materials specifically for people who have been diagnosed with dementia, including opportunities to share your stories. See especially:

- *Persons with Memory Loss,* from the Alzheimer's Association, www.alz.org.
- *I Have Alzheimer Disease,* from the Alzheimer Society of Canada, www.alzheimcr.ca.
- See also the only Web site targeted primarily to patients, www.dasninternational.org.

FOR FAMILY MEMBERS AND CARE PARTNERS

For good, readable overviews of the disease, treatments, and practical advice:

- *Mayo Clinic on Alzheimer's Disease*, by Ronald Petersen, MD, PhD.
- *New Hope for People with Alzheimer's and Their Caregivers*, by Porter Shimer.

For an overall approach helping people with dementia live at the upper limits of their function, intellect, emotion, and spirit:

- *Learning to Speak Alzheimer's: A Groundbreaking Approach for Everyone Dealing with the Disease,* by Joanne Koenig Coste (see summary of the "Principles of Habilitation" at the end of this book).

Caregiver guides that address the emotional stresses of caregiving:

- *Alzheimer's Disease: A Guide for Families,* by Lenore S. Powell with Katie Courtice.
- *Staying Connected While Letting Go: The Paradox of Alzheimer's Caregiving,* by Sandy Braff, MFT, and Mary Rose Olenik.
- *Your Name Is Hughes Hannibal Shanks,* by Lela Knox Shanks. (Shanks combines her personal story with general suggestions. I especially admire the sections "Twenty Coping Strategies" and "The New Life of the Caregiver and Its Rewards.")

For detailed discussions of specific topics (but likely to overwhelm those just beginning to grapple with Alzheimer's):

- *Alzheimer's for Dummies,* by Patricia B. Smith, Mary Mitchell Kenan, and Mark Edwin Kunik, MD, MPH.
- *The Thirty-Six-Hour Day: A Family Guide to Caring for Persons with Alzheimer's Disease, Related Dementing Illness, and Memory Loss in Later Life,* by Nancy Mace, MA, and Peter Rabins, MD.
- For an e-mail–based support group see the "Alzheimer List," hosted at Washington University, St. Louis: alzheimer.wustl.edu/adrc2/alzheimerlist.
- For an online "Caregiver Classroom": www.AlzOnline.net, from the University of Florida. The course on "Positive Caregiving" includes relaxation techniques.

COMMUNICATING

For help as the person with dementia loses communication skills:

- *Steps to Enhancing Communication: Interacting with Persons with Alzheimer's Disease*, brochure from the Alzheimer's Association.
- *Talking to Alzheimer's: Simple Ways to Connect When You Visit with a Family Member or Friend,* by Claudia J. Strauss.

FOR THE CLERGY (BUT NOT JUST CLERGY)

These resources are addressed to clergy but provide a good short introduction for anyone who cares about someone coping with Alzheimer's:

- ❦ *A Guide for Clergy,* a booklet, and *Spirituality and Dementia Care*, a resource list, available from the Alzheimer's Association, www.alz.org/resources.
- ❦ *You Are One of Us: Successful Clergy/Church Connections to Alzheimer's Families*, by Lisa P. Gwyther, published by the Duke University Medical Center.

TAKING CONTROL

It's hard to believe when first coping with the diagnosis, but there are many ways to make a difficult situation more manageable. Most of them require advance planning. It can be a big help, legally and emotionally, to take certain steps while the person with dementia can still participate.

Legal and Financial Planning

Some steps make sense whether or not you face a demanding illness—to give someone a power of attorney (authorizing that person to act for you in business matters if you cannot), to prepare a will, and to review your long-term financial needs.

But Alzheimer's does present some special issues, and it is crucial to seek attorneys and financial advisers who have that expertise. Most chapters of the Alzheimer's Association can suggest well-qualified advisers. A recommendation from another Alzheimer's family is even better.

Helpful resources:

- *Steps to Understanding Financial Issues* and *Steps to Understanding Legal Issues*, brochures from the Alzheimer's Association.
- *Alzheimer's for Dummies*, by Patricia B. Smith, Mary Mitchell Kenan, and Mark Edwin Kunik, MD, MPH, chapters on legal and financial issues.

Health Care Planning

The documents mentioned below are helpful, but it's also important to talk with the people who may have to make health care decisions for you. It eases the difficulty if the patient has suggested some guiding principles.

Health Care Proxy. Who will decide on your medical care if you cannot? It can be crucial to authorize a specific person in writing, especially if the person you choose is not your spouse. A physician or hospital may insist on a formal document naming a health care proxy (also known as a health care agent) before starting treatment. And naming a proxy eliminates one common source of confusion.

Advance Directives (also known as living wills). You may also wish to sign a living will to give your health care proxy some guidance. We chose a general directive not to prolong life in the face of terminal illness, and distributed that document to our physician and our closest family.

Comfort Care, Do Not Resuscitate Orders. When Pete began attending a day program, the director specifically asked for directions how to respond in the event of a heart attack or similar life-threatening emergency. For that we needed a different form, not the living will but one signed by his physician—a "Comfort Care" form, also known as a "Do Not Resuscitate" (DNR) order. Such forms instruct medical staff and emergency workers to administer only "comfort care"—and not, for example, to perform cardiopulmonary resuscitation. The details vary from state to state, but emergency workers may be required to attempt resuscitation unless they have a physician's order to the contrary.

Values History Form. We found the living will too formal to seem very real. The document that helped us discuss the issues was a "Values History Form." This document focuses on what we value in our lives, not on the medical steps that may prolong life or let it go. I was thankful for our discussion at the time, a few years after Pete's diagnosis, and even more so as we made the decision to place Pete in hospice care. You can imagine how comforting it was to re-read his words, "Basically, I don't want to survive forever as a turnip."

Your choices include:

- *Values History Form*, from the Health Sciences Ethics Program, University of New Mexico, Nursing/Pharmacy Building Room 368, Albuquerque, NM 87131, available online at www.unm.edu/~hsethics/valueshist.htm.
- *Handbook for Mortals*, by Joanne Lynn, MD, and Joan Harrold, MD; online edition at www.abcd-caring.org.
- *Five Wishes*, from Aging with Dignity, P.O. Box 1661, Tallahassee FL 32302-1661, www.agingwithdignity.org.

Getting Lost, Wandering, and the Safe Return Program

Some patients get lost because they no longer remember landmarks or directions, and others "wander"—take off on their own—often for no apparent reason, sometimes repeatedly. Many cannot find their way home. The Safe Return Program and its Canadian counterpart, Safely Home, can prevent tragedy. The patient gets a bracelet giving his or her first name, an identifying number, and instructions to call the twenty-four-hour toll-free emergency number. The programs can also fax the patient's photograph and information to the local police.

We were lucky—Pete only took off once and was missing for less than two hours. We didn't think he could have gone far because he had a bad knee and walked slowly—but he turned up five miles away. He'd gotten into a cab. The cabbie realized that his passenger couldn't tell him where to go and took him to a police station. The policeman recognized the bracelet, phoned Safe Return, and brought a cheerful Pete home to his trembling and grateful family.

I could only give thanks I had finally gotten up the nerve to give Pete the Safe Return bracelet. I thought he'd be angry, but once again, I found I'd worried about a problem that wasn't there. He was mildly curious when I put the bracelet on his wrist. That was it.

There had been other times when I lost Pete. The first was at a football game, and luckily we found him soon. But after giving that policeman a description that fit dozens of other alumni flocking to the game, I always carried extra snapshots of Pete in my wallet.

❧ *Safe Return* (brochures in several languages). For details: Alzheimer's Association, www.alz.org/Services.
❧ *Safely Home,* the Alzheimer Society of Canada, www.alzheimer.ca.

CLINICAL TRIALS AND OTHER RESEARCH

Thousands of volunteers—with and without dementia—are needed for ongoing research projects. Many of these projects test potential drugs, but the range of inquiry is great. Current studies needing volunteers here in Boston, for example, include brain imaging, genetic studies, nutrition, tracking specific cognitive changes, testing "brain exercises," and evaluating ways to support families.

We both took part in research projects. It felt great to be contributing, not just coping. It's also a way for friends and relatives who don't have memory issues to join the fight. We are needed for prevention trials, as "control subjects," and for research on normal aging.

Information on current clinical trials and the eligibility requirements are available from the Alzheimer's Association and from ADEAR. The ADEAR Web site, www.alzheimers.org, includes a useful section with questions and answers about Alzheimer's clinical trials.

DONATING YOUR BRAIN

They can have my brain and anything else they want . . . I won't need it.

TERRY, *patient*

My husband, like Terry, wanted to help research as much as he could. Even so, I almost didn't follow through on our plan to donate Pete's brain (also referred to as brain autopsy or tissue donation). It was hard to think about and I wondered if the research center really needed another Alzheimer's brain. But I'm very glad we did go ahead. His illness, which looked so much like Alzheimer's, turned out to be a different dementia, and so his brain continues to teach.

Donating a brain requires advance planning; the research center needs the brain within hours of death. To learn whether there is a brain research center in your area, search the Internet or ask the nearest chapter of the Alzheimer's Association. The center will answer any questions, review its procedures, and ask you to sign some forms. You or your authorized representative can withdraw at any time. Moreover, the family or representative will be asked to confirm or revoke the decision when the brain donor dies.

Most brain centers welcome donations whether or not the deceased has shown signs of dementia—which means that we all have an opportunity to contribute to this research.

For further information, see:

❧ *Alzheimer's for Dummies,* "Considering Brain Donation."

For information on donating organs for transplant, see www. organdonor.gov.

GRIEF

You'd think there would be some books to help patients with grief (as distinct from depression), but I was not able to find any. Thank goodness, there are now some helpful resources for family members:

❧ *Grief and Alzheimer's,* by Doug Manning, an article at www.insightbooks.com, 800-658-9262; also his book *Share My Lonesome Valley: The Slow Grief of Long-Term Care.*

- *Managing Grief and Bereavement: A Guide for Families and Professionals Caring for Memory-Impaired Adults and Other Chronically Ill Persons*, booklet by Edna L. Ballard, Duke Family Support Program, Duke University Medical Center.
- *Staying Connected While Letting Go: The Paradox of Alzheimer's Caregiving*, by Sandy Braff, MFT, and Mary Rose Olenik. Considers the emotional issues through the course of the illness.
- *Matters of Life and Death: Finding the Words to Say Goodbye*, by Carol Wogrin. Directed to a general audience, but includes several Alzheimer's stories.
- *Living with Grief: Alzheimer's Disease*, Hospice Foundation of America, 800-854-3402, www.hospicefoundation.org

In a pioneering caregiver grief study, Dr. Thomas Meuser of Washington University's School of Medicine and Dr. Samuel Marwit of the University of Missouri, St. Louis assess the forms of grief expressed by caregivers. They find significant differences between caregivers who are spouses and those who are adult children, and also variations within these groups that reflect the stage of the patient's illness. See *The Gerontologist,* October 2001 and October 2002 or alzheimer.wustl.edu/adrc2/CGStudy.htm.

End-of-Life Issues

As Pete entered his last chapter, I read and re-read a booklet by Hank Dunn, a hospital chaplain. He includes dementia patients in his thoughtful review of difficult decisions, such as whether to begin or withdraw artificial feeding:

> ❧ *Hard Choices for Loving People: CPR, Artificial Feeding, Comfort Care, and the Patient with Life-Threatening Illness,* by Hank Dunn, A&A Publishers, P.O. Box 1098, Herndon, VA 20172-0174 and www.hardchoices.com.

Hospice

I knew several Alzheimer's families who had used hospice—but only for the last few days of life. It was a surprise to discover that many hospice agencies offer services to dementia patients and their families much sooner. They can provide both practical care and emotional support.

Hospice care focuses on the physical and emotional comfort of the patient with a terminal illness. The setting may be the patient's home or a facility such as an assisted living unit or a nursing home, although some facilities welcome hospice care more readily than others.

Medicare (and some other insurance plans) cover hospice services if the physician certifies that the patient has a terminal illness with a life expectancy of six months or less and meets certain other requirements. The coverage may be extended if the patient continues to meet the eligibility requirements. Coverage is usually available only to those who choose *not* to prolong life by such means as tube feeding.

I knew about the six-month guideline, but couldn't imagine how it would apply to Alzheimer's, where the physical decline is often imperceptibly slow until the last few days or weeks. It didn't even occur to me to ask, although I knew Sunrise, Pete's assisted living facility, was hospitable to hospice care.

Pete had been sick in some unidentifiable way for a few days when I mentioned hospice, almost by accident, to the Sunrise nurse. She jumped at the opening. The hospice nurse came to evaluate Pete two days later. By that evening, hospice had provided a hospital bed for his room at Sunrise and begun twice-daily visits from a home health aide.

I recognized then that the basic steps of Pete's care—keeping him clean, offering him food—had been taking more staff time than I could reasonably expect from an assisted living facility. Hospice staff relieved that burden. Hospice made it possible for Pete to stay with the Sunrise staff who had come to love him, and us, and whom we had come to love. And both Sunrise and hospice were experienced with death in a way that we in the family were not. Their presence and support was a balm to our pain.

It turns out that there are established criteria for applying the six-month guideline to dementia patients. If the dementia patient is no longer ambulatory *and* has medical complications, such as recurrent infections or fevers, or difficulty swallowing or refusing to eat, it may be time to ask whether hospice care is appropriate. But it is wise to research your local hospice agencies well before that point. Some do not provide services to dementia patients, while others invite family members to participate in bereavement groups as soon as they recognize their grief.

For more information:

- *Medicare's Hospice Benefit,* a fact sheet, and *Hospice and Palliative Care in Alzheimer's Disease*, resource list, available from the Alzheimer's Association, www.alz.org/resources.
- *Hospice Foundation of America*, 800-854-3402, 2001 S. St., NW #300, Washington, D.C. 2009. The Web site, www.hospicefoundation.org, offers links to hospice organizations and questions to ask when selecting a hospice.
- *Living with Grief: Alzheimer's Disease,* edited by Kenneth J. Doka, available from the Hospice Foundation of America, discusses issues specific to hospice care for dementia patients.

Words That Helped

The Trying on the Utmost
The Morning it is new
Is Terribler than wearing it
A whole existence through.
—EMILY DICKINSON, FROM "WHILE WE WERE FEARING IT, IT CAME"

The only whole heart is a broken heart.
—UNIDENTIFIED RABBI

I am poured out like water, and all my bones are out of joint;
My heart is like wax, it is melted within my breast.
My strength is dried up like a potsherd . . .
But be not thou far from me, O Lord;
O my strength, make haste to help me.
—PSALM 22

"*Caring for myself is not self-indulgence it is self-preservation*" (quoting *Audre Lorde*). *It's like the instructions they give you on an airplane—put on your own oxygen mask first, then help the person who needs help.*
    —CHRISTIANE NORTHRUP, MD

Thru many troubles, toils, and snares
I have already come;
'Tis grace hath brought me safe thus far,
And grace will lead me home.
    —JOHN NEWTON, "AMAZING GRACE"

The Lord is nigh to the broken hearted; he comforts those who are crushed in spirit.
    —PSALM 34

Ah, when to the heart of man
Was it ever less than a treason
To go with the drift of things,
To yield with a grace to reason,
And bow and accept the end
Of a love or a season?
    —ROBERT FROST, FROM "RELUCTANCE"

Let me not to the marriage of true minds
Admit impediments. Love is not love
Which alters when it alteration finds . . .
Love's not Time's fool, though rosy lips and cheeks
Within his bending sickle's compass come;
Love alters not with his brief hours and weeks,
But bears it out even to the edge of doom. . . .
  —WILLIAM SHAKESPEARE, FROM SONNET 116

I am of the nature to grow old.
There is no way to escape growing old.
I am of the nature to have ill-health.
There is no way to escape ill-health.
I am of the nature to die.
There is no way to escape death.
All that is dear to me and everyone I love
Are of the nature to change.
There is no way to escape being separated from them.
I inherit the results of my actions in body, spirit, and mind.
My actions are the ground on which I stand.
  —THE BUDDHA

Death ends a life, but it does not end a relationship.
—ROBERT ANDERSON, PLAYWRIGHT

Death is strong, but life is stronger.
—REVEREND PHILLIPS BROOKS

To live is so startling, it leaves little time for anything else.
—EMILY DICKINSON

Principles of Habilitation

The "habilitation approach" to Alzheimer's care has now been brought to a worldwide audience with the publication of Joanne Koenig Coste's book, *Learning to Speak Alzheimer's*. Many of us in Massachusetts, however, benefited from an earlier introduction to this approach, pioneered by Joanne and by Paul Raia, PhD, the chapter's director of patient care and family support.

Their teaching makes a dramatic difference. No care partner or professional caregiver is going to succeed all the time, but we can do a great deal to help a person with dementia to live more fully functionally, intellectually, emotionally, and spiritually. In doing so, we ease and enrich our own lives as well.

Here are the core concepts, as summarized in *Learning to Speak Alzheimer's*.

Principles of Habilitation

1. *Make the Physical Environment Work.* Simplify the environment. Accommodate perceptual loss by eliminating distractions.
2. *Know That Communication Remains Possible.* Remember that the emotion behind failing words is far more important than the words themselves and needs to be validated. Although many losses occur with this disease, assume that the patient can still register feelings that matter.
3. *Focus Only on Remaining Skills.* Value what abilities remain. Help the patient compensate for any lost abilities without bringing them to his or her attention.
4. *Live in the Patient's World.* Never question, chastise, or try to reason with the patient. Join her in her current "place" or time, wherever that may be, and find joy with her there.
5. *Enrich the Patient's Life.* Create moments for success; eliminate possible moments of failure, and praise frequently and with sincerity. Attempt to find humor whenever possible.

Acknowledgments

This book began in my oncologist's waiting room, soon after I was diagnosed with cancer. I picked up a little book called *Hope Is Contagious: The Breast Cancer Treatment Survival Handbook,* edited by Margit Esser Porter (Simon & Schuster, 1997). It's a book of short quotations by women who had been through treatment. I read it straight through—at a time when I turned away from all other first-person accounts of the breast cancer experience—and wished we had a similar resource for Alzheimer's.

For turning that idea into a reality, I am especially grateful to the Thursday Alzheimer's support group and to "Writer's II," a work group in the Scholars Program at the Women's Studies Research Center at Brandeis University. Members of both groups gave encouragement, helpful suggestions, and some of the best quotations. Thanks, too, to poet Marguerite Guzmán Bouvard, a resident scholar at the center, for the lines that provide such a perfect epigraph.

Acknowledgments

I wish I could name everyone who has contributed to this book. Those I've quoted are named in the Sources section. I am also grateful to Joyce Cerny, Chris Coffin, Megan Gray, Jeanette Gunther, Sara Holmes, Ann Kiely, Cariadne Margaret Mackenzie, Sam and Barbara Marwit, Tom Meuser, Mitzi Moh, Jeanne Smith, Carol Styczko, Carol Wogrin, and Philip Zaeder for their reviews and suggestions.

Thanks, too, to my agent, Wendy Strothman; to my editor, Marnie Cochran; to the production editor, Erin Sprague; and to George Restrepo who designed the cover.

These people helped me with the book, but I must also thank those who helped us through Alzheimer's. Family and friends: surely you know who you are and how much you meant to us.

Among the professionals to whom I owe everlasting thanks are the leaders of support groups: Stephanie Brett Bell, Barbara Hawley, and Maureen Tardelli at Massachusetts General Hospital; and Ruth Gordon, Joanne Koenig Coste, and Elaine Silverio of the Thursday evening early-onset group. I am also deeply grateful for the work of the Alzheimer's Association and of our outstanding Massachusetts Chapter. My thanks go to all its staff over the years, but especially to Howard Block, Family Advocate; Rachel Hawk, Director of Education; Dr. Paul Raia, Director of Patient Care and Family Support; and James Wessler, President.

Acknowledgments

Among the many kind souls who took care of Pete, special thanks go to Jane Pothier of Hale House in Boston; to Dorothy King, who helped us at home; and to the staff of Sunrise at Gardner Park in Peabody, especially Ann Kiely, Denise Machado Mendonca, and the third-floor caregivers.

And finally, to Nancy Lee and John and Rob: more thanks than I can say, for sharing our family story and for your love and support, far beyond the book.